By David Zinczenko

The Abs Diet
Eat This, Not That! The No-Diet Weight-Loss Solution
Eat This, Not That! For Kids
Eat This, Not That! Supermarket Survival Guide
Eat This, Not That! Restaurant Survival Guide
Eat This, Not That! Best (& Worst) Foods in America!
Cook This, Not That! Kitchen Survival Guide
Cook This, Not That! Skinny Comfort Food
Cook This, Not That! Easy & Awesome 350-Calorie Meals
Grill This, Not That! Backyard Survival Guide
Drink This, Not That! The No-Diet Weight-Loss Solution
Eat This, Not That! No-Diet Diet
The 8-Hour Diet
The New Abs Diet
The New Abs Diet for Women
The New Abs Diet Cookbook
The Abs Diet Eat Right Every Time Guide
The Abs Diet Ultimate Nutrition Handbook
The Abs Diet 6-Minute Meals for 6-Pack Abs
Men, Love & Sex: The Complete User's Guide for Women
Eat It to Beat It!
Eat This, Not That! When You're Expecting
(co-authored with Dr. Jennifer Ashton)
Zero Belly Diet
Zero Belly Cookbook
Zero Belly Smoothies
Zero Belly Breakfasts
Zero Sugar Diet

THE
SUPER
METABOLISM
DIET

BALLANTINE BOOKS
NEW YORK

THE SUPER METABOLISM DIET

The Two-Week Plan to Ignite Your Fat-Burning Furnace and Stay Lean for Life!

DAVID ZINCZENKO

AND KEENAN MAYO

This book proposes a program of diet and exercise recommendations
for the reader to follow. However, you should consult a qualified medical
professional (and, if you are pregnant, your ob/gyn) before starting this or any
other fitness program. Please seek your doctor's advice before making
any decisions that affect your health or extreme changes in your diet, particularly
if you suffer from any medical condition or have any symptom that may
require treatment. As with any diet or exercise program, if at any time you
experience any discomfort, stop immediately and consult your physician.

Published in the United States by Ballantine Books, an imprint of Random House,
a division of Penguin Random House LLC, New York.

BALLANTINE and the HOUSE colophon are registered trademarks of Penguin
Random House LLC.

Some content adapted from EatThis.com, BestLifeOnline.com, and the
Eat This, Not That! book series by David Zinczenko with Matt Goulding.

ISBN 978-1-5247-9662-4
Ebook ISBN 978-1-5247-9663-1

Photographs by Beth Bischoff

Printed in the United States of America on acid-free paper

randomhousebooks.com

First Edition

Book design by Andy Turnbull

*For every American who has bravely battled
one of the single greatest adversaries to our collective
health and well-being: obesity.
Today, you've gained a mighty powerful ally.*

CONTENTS

Introduction

SUPER METABOLISM, SUPER YOU

The Plan That Will Torch Fat and Ignite Your Body's Superpower

W

HAT IF I TOLD you that you have a real life superpower deep inside your body, lying dormant, just waiting to be unleashed? And that once you've activated it, you'll find yourself healthier, happier, smarter, leaner, and more confident than ever before?

Well, it's true. This superpower exists. Discover it, and you'll have a flatter stomach, a toned body, and a longer life—all without sacrificing a thing.

This isn't a dream. It's science. Deep inside your cells there's a biochemical process—a fire, so to speak—that powers your very existence. Without it, your brain wouldn't function, your heart wouldn't beat, your muscles wouldn't twitch. Its magic— this mysterious, energy-churning life force—actually means the difference between having the lean, strong body of your dreams, and trudging woefully through your days saddled with the burden of unwanted weight. Your superpower also means the difference between feeling okay, feeling energetic, and feeling flat-out *amazing*. But best of all? Once you've activated your superpower, it will do *all of the hard work* for you.

Imagine a world in which you didn't have to torture yourself at the gym for hours on end. Imagine a world in which you didn't have to slash tons of calories from your diet. Imagine a world where you don't feel guilty every time you indulge in your favorite tasty foods—or desperately follow some newfangled dieting fad. Imagine a world in which you only have to . . . *activate your superpower.*

I know, I sound like the movie trailer voiceover guy—you know, *"Imagine a world where civilizations fall, and heroes must rise . . ."* But this introduction is the trailer for a new you.

And guess what?

In this story, you're the hero.

Because you have this power inside you right now. And *The Super Metabolism Diet* will help you find it.

Still, I'm guessing you don't feel much like a hero yet. There's a really good chance that your metabolism isn't exactly firing at full speed. *Right now, 155 million Americans are overweight.*

If you're one of them, or if you're feeling stressed out and depressed, or sapped of energy at all times, I'm here to turn that barely flickering light into a burning star. And, with the science-backed contents of *The Super Metabolism Diet* as your guide, you'll finally achieve your body's most powerful fat-burning potential. Best of all, you'll be bulletproofing your body against the harsh forces of age—and worse. According to David Mangelsdorf, PhD, a noted metabolism expert at the University of Texas Southwestern, everything you're doing to harm your metabolism does more than just affect your waist size.

"Each one of the things that you're doing is a risk factor for more than just burning energy and getting fat," he says. "You're at risk of disease."

Now, the top scientists—many of whom I've spoken to for this book—haven't discovered a magical switch for your metabolism just yet, but they have indeed begun uncovering more and more about how it works and what it means. And I can tell you this: Gaining control of your body is far easier—and far more attainable—than you ever imagined. Yes, you *can* be forty years old and have the metabolism of someone fifteen years younger overnight (okay, two weeks!). You just need to understand the key drivers and elemental makeup of your inner superpower.

Your metabolism is a dizzyingly complex process deep inside your cells that takes the food you eat and either stores it as fat, muscle, and other bodily matter, or burns it off as energy. And everything in my plan is designed to get your body doing a lot more burning and a lot less storing.

Your superpower needs the right fuel to thrive—and needs to be fed properly. Stress and lack of proper sleep are both major metabolism killers. So is that Netflix binge. And when your hormones—your body's inner organ-to-organ radio network—fail to communicate properly, your metabolism takes a severe beating, as well. You'll learn about all of these wretched metabolic supervillains in *The Super Metabolism Diet,* as well as all of the easy ways you can combat them—and defeat them—head-on.

But the very foundation of your metabolism is, of course, your diet. If you eat the right foods—and choose to embrace the Super Metabolism Movement Plan—you'll find yourself shedding extra pounds, feeling happier, and bursting with life.

The wrong foods?

Well, let's just say they're your very own Kryptonite.

Believe me, I know.

Like so many American males raised in the 1970s and '80s, by the time I reached young adulthood in the late '80s I knew a few irrefutable truths. Among them: Michael Jordan was a god, Brooke Shields was a goddess, and fat, of course, was the devil. After all, this was the era in which the "Food Guide Pyramid" was slapped on elementary school walls in between pictures of George Washington and Harriet Tubman, and it instructed kids to load up on upward of *eleven servings* of bread and other grains every single day as the very foundation of a healthy diet. High-fat foods—fish, meats, and dairy—were near the top of the pyramid as major no-no's, right beneath cake and Coca-Cola. It's no wonder Americans at the time were watching their waistlines balloon at an extraordinary rate. By 1990, more than one in 10 American adults was obese.

Don't think for a minute that I'm making light of this. I was among them. In my younger years in Pennsylvania, I was well acquainted with terms like "husky," "full-bodied," and "big-boned." Thirty years later, I'll say it in bright, clear language: I was chunky. And I knew as well as anyone what it was like to weigh in on the heavier side of your peer group. When it came to eating, I made every single mistake you could possibly make. My best friends? Yes, there were Bob, Scott, and Dean. But there were also Little Debbie, Baby Ruth, and both Mike and Ike. By the time I was fourteen years old, I had packed more than two hundred pounds on an otherwise slender, five-foot-ten frame.

Like any impressionable kid, I took after my father, who was more than one hundred pounds overweight for much of his adult life and suffered through all of the ailments that plague men who carry the harsh burden of such weight. First there was the hypertension, then the diabetes. Eventually, there was the heart attack. Often getting out of chairs and climbing the stairs proved to be difficult tasks. Unfortunately, he ignored many of the telltale signs about his health, and his life was cut short too soon after a stroke at the age of fifty-two.

I, on the other hand, chose a different path. Joining the Navy Reserves after college, I finally shed all of those unwanted pounds—thank you, boot camp—and I went on to a career as the head of *Men's Health, Women's Health,* and *Prevention* for many years and then *Men's Fitness.* In 2013, I launched my own company, called Galvanized Media, which publishes Eat This, Not That!, Best Life, Zero Belly, and other products that redefine the new era of healthy living. As the name of my company attests, I've dedicated my life to the pursuit of helping people understand the importance of proper nutrition and the dangers of carrying around too much weight.

Today, all of those years of young adulthood still weigh heavily on my memory. I've always wondered: Why do some people work so hard to achieve the body of the dreams but continually fall short, while others will put in a fraction of their effort and yet walk through life with the physique of Jennifer Lawrence or Chris Hemsworth?

Deep down, I've discovered, it all has to do with your metabolism.

We've come a long way in our understanding of the complexity of our metabolisms and the role it plays in weight loss. For instance, we've learned that even so-called healthy people cause damage to their metabolisms every day. In 2016, in fact, researchers revealed the findings of a six-year study of candidates from TV's blockbuster fat-loss show, *The Biggest Loser.* They tracked sixteen candidates who lost literally hundreds of pounds through rigorous diet and fitness regimens. Losing all of that weight was great, right? Even *inspiring*?

Well, wrong, actually. Though I'll admit that it makes for great TV watching someone suffer through the misery of military-style fitness and the agony of crash dieting, as the researchers revealed, those weight-loss contestants ended up cutting so many calories from their diets that they emerged from the ordeal with their metabolisms likely irreparably damaged.

Talk about shooting yourself—and your superpower—in the foot.

A FULL SEMESTER'S WORTH OF BIOCHEMISTRY 101 IN 80 WORDS!

In your cells, your metabolism operates by doing two things simultaneously: it builds up tissue, such as fat—a process called anabolism—and breaks things down to create adenosine triphosphate (ATP, or energy). That process, meanwhile, is called catabolism. Combined it's called the CTA cycle, and it's essentially your body's inner power plant. In the simplest terms, your body weight is the result of your anabolism, the energy your body builds up, subtracted from catabolism, the energy your body releases.

Those contestants aren't the only ones in America taking things to extremes in pursuit of weight loss. After all, we've become a nation divided on just about everything—whether it's politics, football, *or* food. As I just mentioned, fat was the food-world bogeyman for a generation. Today? Courtesy of the Paleo, the Ketogenic Diet, and other fashionable dieting movements, it's carbs. As a culture, we drop entire macronutrients from our diets more often than Kanye West drops new pairs of Yeezys.

And, frankly, I couldn't sit by any longer as I watched our collective health continue to deteriorate. Today, we've come a long way from 1990—and entirely in the wrong direction. Right now, according to the latest figures from the Centers for Disease Control and Prevention, 36.5 percent of all Americans are obese, which represents a 25 percent increase from the high-flying low-fat days of the first Bush administration. If you're also counting simply "overweight" people—or those with a body mass index (BMI) of between 25 and 30—that figure expands to a staggering 68.8 percent. Oh, and speaking of body mass: Since 2001, we've collectively experienced a tenfold increase. The American Diabetes Association's most recent figures says that 29.1 million Americans—or just under 10 percent of the entire country—suffer from diabetes, with 1.4 million new cases emerging every single year!

Here's the deal: If you want to effectuate real, meaningful change in your life, you needn't starve yourself or log six hours of gym time every single day. You don't need to torture yourself emotionally and put on a hair shirt every time you crave a dessert or your favorite burger. You don't have to log two-a-days at the gym and guzzle protein shakes on the hour. Success is actually much, much easier, and it's achieved by unleashing your own inner superpower and letting it do all of the hard work for you.

How exactly do you do it? On the Super Metabolism Diet:

- You'll eat delicious foods!
- You'll move more, building strength and burning more energy!
- You'll relax and recharge!
- And you'll never ever feel hungry!

That's right: This is a diet in which you don't actually, well . . . "diet." I know that seems a little puzzling, and I wouldn't be surprised if you took a moment and quietly eyed the jacket cover to ensure you didn't pick up the wrong book by mistake. But it's true: I want you to eat—a lot. Which is, I'd argue, why this is actually the *best* diet of all.

By now you've probably heard one of today's leading workplace clichés: "Work smarter, not harder." Well, consider this book the physical manifestation of "Eat smarter, not less."

That's why this diet includes three full meals a day and a tasty snack. The focus of *The Super Metabolism Diet* is rooted in getting the best foods that any neighborhood grocery store has to offer. And all it takes is fourteen days.

You'll enjoy delicious Super Proteins—including in your mornings. What are Super Proteins, you ask? They're the crucial, flubber-frying muscle builders that will not only kick-start your metabolism but they'll also perform double duty, as your body will actually *burn energy* while you digest them. (Yes, win-win.)

Then you'll be getting more Super Fats—the special ones filled with nutrients that increase satiety, protect you from heart disease, and come packed with free-radical fighting antioxidants. And there are Super Carbs. Yes, you can eat your favorite carbs, just so long as you stick to the ones on my list—several delicious magic bullets for weight loss—which come packed with plenty of fiber.

In addition to eating great-tasting foods, you're going to learn not only about all of the lifestyle forces that have a direct influence on your metabolic processes—chiefly sleep and stress—but I'm also going to offer handy and super-easy, actionable guides for ensuring that you're getting more rest and feeling less stressed than you have in years.

Finally, yes: I'm going to ask you to exercise. No, it's not essential, and no, I'm not asking you to sign up for your nearest marathon or mud run. Frankly, I'm not even going to ask you to pony up for a gym membership. As you'll discover in these pages, if you have four limbs, five minutes, and a rudimentary understanding of the laws of gravity, you're already fully equipped with all of the muscle-maintaining and muscle-building tools anyone can ever need. And when you reach the Super Metabolism Movement Plan, you'll discover a largely unreported and utterly remarkable piece of cutting-edge scientific research that will change the way that you look at your body—and your metabolism—forever. (Hint: When it comes to losing weight, simply moving around—not even exercising—plays a greater role in activating your body's energy-burning engines than you ever imagined.)

Now, are you ready to get started? Good, because it's your movie, hero.

Let the cameras roll.

THE *SUPER METABOLISM* DIET AT A GLANCE

HERE'S A HELPFUL snapshot of *The Super Metabolism Diet,* the two-week guide to optimize your body's natural fat-burning apparatus and keep it stoked for life.

The *Super Metabolism* Pillars:	**S**uper Proteins, Super Carbs, and Super Fats
	Upping Your Energy Expenditure
	Power Snacks
	Essential Calories, Vitamins, and Minerals
	Relaxing and Recharging

MEALS

● Eat three square meals a day, plus one snack.

STAY FLUID

● You'll be maximizing your daily intake of the simplest and most plentiful resource on the planet: water!

PACK IN YOUR NUTRIENTS

All meals contain these key ingredients:

SUPER PROTEINS

● Eggs, salmon, lean beef, and more.

SUPER CARBS

● Oatmeal, whole wheat, quinoa, and more.

SUPER FATS

● Avocados, nut butters, olive oil, and more.

SUPER SNACKS

● Yogurt, carrots, hummus, and more.

SUPER FRIENDS

● Tea, spices, and more.

ELIMINATE DIETARY SUPERVILLAINS

● Breads and cereals (that aren't mentioned in Super Carbs; see page 18)
● Saturated fats (except lean beef and some dairy)
● Alcohol (particularly beer and mixed drinks)
● Refined carbohydrates
● High-fructose corn syrup
● Sodas

ELIMINATE LIFESTYLE SUPERVILLAINS

- Conquer your stress.
- Maximize your sleep.
- Avoid unnecessary chemicals.

ADOPT SUPER-SMART STRATEGIES

- Be aware of every bite!
- Eat carbs at night.
- Boost your protein—especially at breakfast!
- Make your food spicy and tasty and interesting!
- Embrace the magic elixir of tea.
- Cheat! Cheat! Cheat!

MOVE, MOVE, MOVE!

A strong metabolism means you need to be more active. Here are three tiers involved in the Super Metabolism Movement Plan:

TIER ONE
GET RESTLESS!
Take walks, climb stairs, stand and sit, and even fidget!

TIER TWO
BUILD YOUR BODY (OPTIONAL)
Engage in strength training for muscle maintenance and growth.

TIER THREE
UP YOUR EFFICIENCY (OPTIONAL)
Elevate your workouts by adding intensity.

Chapter 1

LIGHT YOUR FIRE, CHANGE YOUR LIFE

Six Ways Turbocharging Your Metabolism Will Dramatically Improve How You Look, Feel, and Live

IF WE ASKED the average American to write down the superpower of his or her dreams, I'd wager Hugh Jackman's last *Wolverine* paycheck that it wouldn't be "shooting cobwebs from my wrists," "having retractable bone claws," or even necessarily "having the ability to fly." It wouldn't be wielding Wonder Woman's golden "lasso of truth" or having Catwoman's ability to sneak anywhere she wants to go, either.

No, as much as we all love comic book movies—and we all, deep down, dream of wearing a cape and darting across rooftops to fight crime—it's safe to say that the superpower we'd want most is to be able to improve and better our minds and bodies at will—and that means being able to successfully lose weight, easily and efficiently, and stay lean for life.

You don't have to take it from me! Simply look at the facts: Right now, the self-help industry is valued at $13 billion annually and is only expected to grow exponentially in the years ahead.

But for all of the books, apps, life coaches and gurus, and seminars and workshops we're willing to shell out our hard-earned money for—to boost our productivity, bolster our confidence, find balance and happiness, be more active, de-stress and decompress, and razor-sharpen our intelligence and cognitive cunning—I'm continually astonished by how we can't see the forest for the trees.

Here's the truth: If you unleash the full force of your metabolism, you'll improve in literally *all* of those areas.

It's true! Your metabolism is the tide that lifts all boats. And trust me: Once you've ignited it and your body transforms into a more efficient, fat-melting machine, you'll be floored by how its fire will echo through literally all of the facets of your life.

Here are just some of the ways a fully functioning metabolism will be a force for good in your life:

You'll Lose Weight Effortlessly— and Keep It Off

WHEN YOU'VE devoted your entire professional career to helping Americans lead healthier, more fulfilling lives (and you are a health and wellness contributor to *The Today Show*), you find that a lot of people will approach you in odd places with a single question in mind: "What's the best way to lose weight?"

Without fail, it always pains me to see their disappointment— in a Starbucks line or at the gym—when I give them the truth: "It's not just one thing."

To be sure, I'm not dodging the question like a politician's press secretary, and it doesn't mean weight loss isn't easily achieved with the right plan and a healthy sense of determination. It just means that the mechanics of weight loss are slightly more complicated that most of us would like to believe.

But those who can lose weight have one thing in common: a healthy metabolism.

When you've got a fully optimized metabolism, not only will you have harnessed the full power of Mother Nature's fat-burning mechanism—after all, everything in my plan is designed so that your body burns more energy and stores less fat than it did before—but you'll also be adopting new habits that will bolster your weight-loss efforts. A fully functioning fuel furnace means you will have a supercharging effect on *all* of the many weight-loss factors: sleep, stress, energy levels, and more. You'll be eating more, moving more, and avoiding all of the toxic obstacles in modern life that affect your metabolism in negative ways.

And because *The Super Metabolism Diet* doesn't torture you—and you can indeed eat basically all of your favorite, delicious foods—it's easy to maintain.

But, like I said, it's not just *one thing*. You're going to need to eat the right foods, *enough* of the right foods, and I'd urge you to adopt the movement plan contained in this book.

If you do, you'll see a change not only in your body but also in the way you view the world.

You'll Be Supersmart

EVERYONE HAS their favorite childhood game. For some, it's Candy Land. For others, it's Chutes and Ladders. For me? That's easy: It was Hungry Hungry Hippos.

The game involves nothing more than a board, four plastic

hippos with working mouths controlled by four players, and a bunch of marbles that get chomped faster than a cake at a four-year-old's birthday party.

Now, if the major organs of your body—your heart, your liver, your brain, your lungs—were playing this game among themselves for the stuff contained in your food, my guess is you'd probably think that your heart would win. After all, it's got to pump a *lot* of blood—your average adult heart moves five quarts of blood every minute, or roughly two thousand gallons every day—to keep you alive. It's also the only organ you can actually hear working, thumping along in your chest like a bass drum. Surely your strong heart needs the most fuel, right?

Almost, but not quite.

The answer? Drumroll, please . . .

It's the gooey mass sitting right behind your eyes: your brain.

In fact, if your brain were playing Hungry Hungry Hippos, it would probably swallow up more than marbles. It's so hungry it would chomp up your entire board.

If you're at rest—say, lying on the couch—your brain is responsible for roughly a third of your entire calorie burn. After all, we humans didn't rise to the top of the food chain because we have the strength of a lion, the speed of a cheetah, or the ferocity of a bear. No, we're the head honchos on this planet because of our intelligence and savvy problem-solving skills. And that cognition doesn't happen just by magic. We have to feed it with the right fuel. I hate to be a downer, but if you were to cut off your brain's supply of food, you'd instantly lose consciousness and eventually fall into a coma and die.

If you're not eating the right foods, not only are you doing your body a disservice—and piling on the pounds around your midsection—you're actually making yourself dumber. Study after study has shown that people suffering from diabetes are far more likely to suffer a decline in cognitive function—and even experience dementia—than people who don't have diabetes.

According to researchers at the Brigham and Women's Hospital at Harvard University, your diet directly influences your memory, and poor eating decisions—chiefly a diet loaded with saturated and trans fats—can help kick-start the insidious onset of dementia as you advance in years. Those harmful ingredients will boost the amount of low-density lipoprotein (LDL) cholesterol in your bloodstream, while also exacerbating the spread of beta-amyloid plaques on the brain—which are "sticky protein clusters" that are one of the chief culprits in Alzheimer's disease.

"We know [diets high in cholesterol and saturated fats are] bad for your heart," wrote Francine Grodstein, associate professor of medicine at Harvard Medical School and epidemiologist at Brigham and Women's Hospital. "There is now a lot of evidence that it's also bad for your brain."

But if you're feeding your metabolism, you're actually feeding your brain, too—and many of the foods found in the diet contained in this book double as awesome brain boosters, such as . . .

LEAN BEEF. Swiss researchers discovered that of three different breakfast types—high-carbohydrate, high-protein, and a balance of both—the high-protein meal helped men score better on a computer memory test (similar to the electronic game Simon). "Short-term memory can be better after a protein-rich meal because the food increases your levels of the amino acids tyrosine and phenylalanine," says Karina Fischer, PhD, the study's lead author.

SPINACH AND OTHER LEAFY GREENS. Dark or leafy greens contain high levels of folate and vitamin B_{12}, which may protect the brain against dementia. Researchers from Tufts and Boston universities observed subjects in the famous Framingham Heart Study and found those with high levels of homocysteine had nearly double the risk of developing Alzheimer's disease. High

SOAK IN THOSE A.M. RAYS!

Stepping outside in the morning could help you finally shed excess pounds. Researchers at Northwestern University's Feinberg School of Medicine found that individuals who were exposed to early morning sunlight (not later in the day) had lower body mass indexes (BMIs) independent of other factors known to affect metabolism, like exercise, calorie consumption, or age. Don't forget your sunscreen, though!

homocysteine is associated with low levels of folate and vitamins B_6 and B_{12}, leading researchers to speculate that getting more B vitamins may be protective.

BLUEBERRIES. Dark-colored fruits and vegetables, especially blueberries, strawberries, and spinach, are high in antioxidants. In research on rats at the USDA Human Nutrition Research Center on Aging at Tufts University, James Joseph, PhD, found that older rats fed blueberry extract had improved short-term memory and motor skills.

OATMEAL. University of Toronto researchers recently determined that eating carbohydrate-rich foods like oatmeal is equivalent to a shot of glucose, a.k.a. blood sugar, injected into your brain. According to the study, the higher the concentration of glucose in your blood, the better your memory and concentration.

The truth is that your brain requires a steady stream of glucose at all times in order to keep your synapses and neurons firing properly. Ultimately, your brain needs sugar (the natural kind accompanied by fiber). It also needs a steady stream of fatty acids and micronutrients such as B vitamins, iron, magnesium, niacin, and the compound lipoic acid. In the diet plan contained in this book, you'll find all of the delicious ways of getting these ingredients every day.

You'll Be Happier and Less Depressed

IF YOU'VE EVER found yourself scraping the bottom of a tub of ice cream after a bad day, you already know that your emotions can influence what you eat. But what you may not realize is that what you eat can dramatically alter your mental health. In other words: There's a direct connection between "mood and food."

Simple food choices can make the difference between feeling worse and feeling more stable, says research from a February 2015 study by Virginia Tech College of Agriculture and Life Sciences. Eighteen percent of the population suffers some form of anxiety disorder, and 6.7 percent of the American population over the age of eighteen has been diagnosed with clinical depression.

You don't have to be officially diagnosed (many people aren't, anyway) to know what an overwhelming burden it can be when you are even marginally anxious or depressed. It's a simple fact: The foods we consume can play a major role in increasing the frequency, depth, and duration of bouts of depression or anxiety, especially if we're already predisposed to experiencing them.

According to a landmark Spanish study published in *PLOS One*, eating the wrong fats is unfortunately one of the surefire ways to find yourself depressed. The researchers studied 12,059 men and women over the course of several years and discovered that those with a diet high in trans fats—or 1.5 grams daily, to be more specific (or about the same amount found in a Whopper from Burger King)—were 48 percent more likely to experience heightened levels of the blues. And, if you're depressed, you're 58 percent more at risk of obesity.

On the flipside, boosting your intake of the right fruits and vegetables—the very same fruits and vegetables you'll find in *The Super Metabolism Diet*—will indeed give you a sunnier outlook on life. According to a 2016 study published in the *American Journal of Public Health,* researchers poured over the eating habits of 12,385 Australian adults over the course of three years and found that "increased fruit and vegetable consumption was predictive of increased happiness, life satisfaction, and well-being." Furthermore, the study authors reported that those healthier eaters upped their "satisfaction points" by "0.24, which is equal in size to the psychological gain of moving from unemployment to employment."

In other words, simply eating better foods will make you as happy as scoring a new job!

In the past, scientists weren't sure why depression, diabetes, and dementia seemed to cluster in epidemiological studies or why having one of these health issues increases your risk for the others. But in a study published in the journal *Diabetologia*, researchers have found that when blood glucose levels are elevated (more on that later), levels of a protein that encourages the growth of neurons and synapses drops. Translation: The simple act of eating way too much sugar makes your brain work at a suboptimal level.

In addition to spiking your insulin—something you'll be avoiding on the Super Metabolism Diet—too much sugar leads to inflammatory bodies spreading throughout your noggin and promotes oxidative stress, the scenario in which our natural defenses against your body's natural (and harmful) free radicals prove to be insufficient. According to the landmark Framingham Heart Study, which tested 2,828 people over the course of many years, oxidative stress is directly linked to obesity.

Meanwhile, studies have shown that when you eat a diet based on the right fruits, vegetables, fats, and carbohydrates—all crucial ingredients you'll find in the diet I've laid out in this book—you're essentially attacking oxidative stress head-on. In a matter of only days, you'll notice an acute change in the way you feel.

You'll Be Super Productive— and Make More Money

TOMATO TIMERS. To-do lists. Email reminders. Standing desks. More music. Less music. Do-your-most-difficult-task-first-thing-in-the-morning. For all the "productivity hacks" that millions upon millions of working people swear by, it always pains me that the vast majority of us miss the absolute biggest one of all: your diet. (If you're skeptical, try to remember the last time you accomplished anything meaningful on an empty stomach.)

Yet when you think about all of the things that contribute to getting things done, you rarely hear people giving credit where credit is due. It all starts the moment you put food into your mouth and swallow.

As I'll explain in depth in this book, if you're eating too many overly sugary and processed foods—that means everything from bottles of Coca-Cola to high-sugar cereals and dishes piled high with pasta—you'll get a surge of energy followed by an ugly crash. And if you're eating *ultra-high-fat* meals—think of too much sausage in the morning or a big greasy steak or grisly cheeseburger in the afternoon—you're actually overloading your digestive system, which means that your brain function hobbles and you get drowsy.

Having a sluggish metabolism and dragging yourself through your working hours isn't exactly the same as boarding a rocket-ship to the corner office of your dreams. In fact, quite the opposite. According to a study published in the *Journal of Occupational and Environmental Medicine* in 2014, the adverse health effects of obesity in American workers lead to missed workdays that costs states $8.65 billion per year. The study suggests that "reduced productivity" from poor health costs are even higher.

But when you adopt the eating plan I've laid out here, your body will become a more efficient energy burner. And when that happens, you'll find that you're a more energetic person, too. As I mentioned before, boosting your intake of fruits and vegetables will give you a cognitive edge. Well, the same goes for many of the Super Proteins, Super Fats, and Super Carbs contained in this book. Take tuna, for instance.

A serving of tuna contains 69 percent of your daily dose of vitamin B_6, which according to a number of studies, is linked to motivation. That's because lacking B_6 leads to feelings of depression—and when we're not feeling quite like ourselves, it's harder to be productive. And there are other benefits. In a study conducted at the University of Maryland Medical Center, researchers were able to use the essential vitamin to both prevent and treat attention-deficit-hyperactivity disorder, more often known as ADHD. The common disorder is known to increase levels of inattention, hyperactivity, and impulsivity—all traits that are needed to have a productive day.

You'll Be Sexier—and Better at Sex

"CONFIDENCE."

It's an old joke in the magazine world. In over two decades of being an editor, I noticed a trend: Whenever my writers ask a beautiful woman (or man) what qualities she found most seductive in a partner, the answer is inevitably the most cliché of all clichés . . . "confidence." And when you've edited as many stories as I have about sex and relationships (literally thousands), you find yourself fantasizing about a Hollywood ingénue who will answer the question with anything else. But no, it was never "V-cut abs," "tight blue jeans," or "scruff."

It's always, simply, "confidence."

Now, let's set aside unoriginality and focus on the truth: Confidence makes you a magnet for the opposite sex—whether you're a man or a woman—and you can pretty much draw a straight line between your fully charged metabolism and the self-assurance with which you walk through the world.

When you're eating for your metabolism, your food choices will be evident in your waistline, your mood, your energy levels, and your appearance (particularly your skin and hair). And get this: Certain foods also play a role in your attractiveness in a much more immediate way—I'm talking about food's effect on pheromones: the chemicals we excrete in our sweat, saliva, and other body fluids that have a social or sexual effect. (For proof, see the sidebar "Super Metabolism After Dark" on page 12.)

Also, when your metabolism is ignited and you're a more efficient fuel burner, you'll have:

> **Increased stamina.** It's simply a fact: When you have higher energy levels, stronger muscles, and more oxygen—and blood!—flowing through you veins, you'll find that you can bump-'n'-grind for far longer than ever before. And, as you'll soon discover, certain ingredients in the Super Metabolism Diet are all but guaranteed to boost your sexual stamina.

Consider the humble apple. If you knew what it contained, you probably would've thought twice before giving one to your high school teacher. This everyday fruit contains high levels of quercetin, an antioxidant flavonoid that has been found to play a role in improving endurance. According to Nashville-based nutritionist Sarah-Jane Bedwell, RD, LDN, quercetin "can help to create new mitochondria in the body's cells and increase one's oxidative capacity." As I'll explain, more mitochondria directly equals a stronger metabolism.

> **Better erections.** If you're overweight, you're clogging the arteries that send blood from your heart to your penis. It's something all too many men know all too well. According to the Cleveland Clinic Center for Continuing Education, 40 percent of men forty years in age (or older) are afflicted by erectile dysfunction (ED).

Let me be clear: A slower metabolism means more fat. And

SUPER METABOLISM AFTER DARK

Yes, by eating certain foods, we can all boost our sex appeal
(through the release of certain hormones that may attract others),
increase our blood flow, and experience new endorphin highs.
Herewith I've included your ultimate sex-minded shopping list that
can be found in any supermarket or restaurant.

FATTY FISH Omega-3 fatty acids not only benefit your heart but
also raise dopamine levels in the brain. This spike in dopamine improves
circulation and blood flow, triggering arousal. "Dopamine will make you
feel more relaxed and connected to your partner, which makes sex
more fun," says psychotherapist Tammy Nelson, PhD. Just make sure
you buy the right kind. (Hint: It rhymes with "Talmon" or "Suna.")

EGGS For men, the boosting ingredient in eggs is choline, a natural
chemical that burns fat and helps set his pants afire. Choline triggers
the production of nitric oxide (NO), which relaxes arteries in the penis
and enables better blood flow.

HOT SAUCE A recent study from France found men who have a
taste for spicy foods tend to have higher testosterone levels than those
who can't handle the heat. In both men and women, peppers help
stimulate those super pleasurable endorphins!

CELERY It turns out celery, of all things, is one seriously sexy stalk,
containing androsterone, a male sex pheromone released through
perspiration.

GREEN TEA The brew is rich in compounds called catechins, which
have been shown to blast away belly fat and speed the liver's capacity
for turning fat into energy. But that's not all: Catechins also boost desire
by promoting blood flow to your nether region. Blood flow to the
genitals = feeling of sexual excitement, so sipping the stuff will, well,
make you want to get it on.

DARK CHOCOLATE There's a reason chocolate became a gift given before amorous activity. Cacao increases levels of the mood-boosting hormone serotonin, which can lower stress levels, boosting desire and making it easier to reach orgasm. And that's not all: Cocoa also increases blood flow through the arteries and relaxes blood vessels, sending blood to all the right regions, which can boost sexual pleasure.

SPINACH "Spinach is rich in magnesium, a mineral that decreases inflammation in blood vessels, increasing blood flow," explains Cassie Bjork, RD, LD, of Healthy Simple Life. "Increased blood flow drives blood to the extremities, which, like Viagra, can increase arousal and make sex more pleasurable," says Nelson. "Women will find it is easier to have an orgasm, and men will find that erections come more naturally."

LEAN BEEF One of the causes of fatigue in women is iron deficiency. The condition can sap energy, which may result in a low sex drive. "Iron deficiency is common and can result in feelings of exhaustion, weakness and irritability, which doesn't make anyone feel like getting intimate," says Bjork. Iron-rich lean beef will rev her engine and get her feeling sexy again!

when your blood vessels become clogged with the nasty side effects—such as plaque formation on your arteries—you're looking at a smaller expressway from your heart to your member. And slower blood flow means weaker erections.

> **Greater hormonal balance.** As you'll learn, the hormone cortisol—also known as your stress hormone—plays a major role in both your metabolism and your sex drive and sexual execution. If you're a man, cortisol is directly related to erectile dysfunction. If you're a woman, studies show that heightened levels of cortisol means less sexual arousal. When you're on the Super Metabolism Diet—and feeling better and sleeping better and feeling less stressed—you'll find that your cortisol levels will be entirely under control.

As far as I'm concerned, we're in the middle of a countrywide sex crisis. A study published in March 2017 in the journal *Archives of Sexual Behavior* contained some truly depressing stats: Americans are having measurably less sex than they used to. As of 2014, married couples are down to fifty-six times a year (from sixty-seven in 1989), and Millennials—yes, the Tinder-swiping generation—aren't exactly pulling their weight in the bedroom, either. In fact, they're having sex less often than the previous generation. "The results suggest that Americans are having sex less frequently due to two primary factors," write the researchers, "an increasing number of individuals without a steady or marital partner and a decline in sexual frequency among those with a partner." That's right: married people and single people are having less sex.

If you follow the diet contained in this book, you'll boost your chances of not being one of them.

You'll Look and Feel Younger

IT'S IMPORTANT TO take control now, because your metabolism peaks in your early twenties and slows itself down at a pace of around 2 percent every decade. According to some experts' calculations, your body burns 200 fewer calories per day in your mid-forties than it did in your mid-twenties. That means that if you didn't change anything about your eating habits or adjust your behavior in the slightest, you'd be gaining upward of twenty pounds a year!

When your metabolism starts to sputter, it sets in motion a ghastly cycle, beginning when you become less active. When you become less active, you lose muscle mass. When you lose muscle mass, your metabolism slows because having less muscle mass means you're burning fewer and fewer calories. After all, your muscles are your metabolic superstars—they're a hotbed of your mitochondria, the tiny hardworking organelles in your cells that are largely responsible for turning the substrates stripped from the food you eat into adenosine triphosphate (ATP), the scientific term for energy.

When you reach your thirties, you produce less human growth hormone—which helps your body grow and maintain your organs and tissues—which makes it even harder for you to gain back that muscle. Your thyroid starts producing less thyroid hormones (chiefly T3 and T4), which regulate metabolism, appetite, your heart beat, thermogenesis (or the production of heat), and muscle function, among other important duties. If you're a man, you've got less muscle-building, energy-producing testosterone. If you're a woman, you have less estrogen. And as you approach your menopausal years, your energy-producing hormones plummet. And because your body has an inherently worse muscle-to-fat ratio than a man of the same age and size, you're burning less energy.

Without you even realizing it, your body spirals into a "vicious cycle" that mirrors the experience that anyone suffering from addiction knows all too well: Cravings lead to a drug, which leads to guilt, which leads to pain, which leads to more cravings, and so on. In the case of your metabolism, having less energy means you have less muscle mass, which leads to a slower resting metabolic rate, which leads to less energy, and the cycle continues.

According to a National Health and Nutrition Examination Survey that polled adults between the ages of twenty-five and forty-four, the male subjects gained between 3 and 4 percent of their body weight every ten years, while females gained more than 5 percent. Additionally, the rate at which men experience more rapid metabolic decline begins at forty years of age, and for women at fifty. According to researchers at Johns Hopkins University, the average adult can expect to gain roughly one to two pounds every year "from early adulthood until middle age." And the Centers for

Disease Control and Prevention say that people in their sixth decade and up are far likelier to be obese than their younger counterparts.

Why does this happen? Why are the cruel forces of nature so stacked against our waistlines?

Well, there's an inflection point in every person's life when he or she goes from *growing* as a human organism to simply maintaining, or aging. I'm sorry for the tough love, but such is life. But good news! The Super Metabolism Diet is scientifically designed to serve as a bulwark against the cruel forces of age. Once you're eating for your body's fat-burning mechanism, you'll look and feel more youthful than you've felt in years.

And if you want to combat the forces of age—which, in fitness terms, is entirely possible—I've got you covered. I've included in this book a trove of amazing exercises that will not only keep your metabolism burning hot but will also improve your body's oxygen-consuming apparatus and will make you a far more efficient and healthy fat-burner. In effect, you'll be doing the equivalent of turning back the clock with your finger.

But it all begins with the foods you put into your body.

IT'S A BIG WORLD, AFTER ALL . . .

Yes, and it's all thanks to our sluggish metabolisms. Consider this: According to recent estimates, Americans fork out roughly $210 billion annually directly on obesity-related health issues—which translates to 21 percent of all healthcare spending! Our exploding waistlines don't just affect the afflicted—no, it affects the everyday lives of everyone. Here are just a few ways in which we're accounting for our weight gain.

SUPER AMBULANCES According to the American Ambulance Association, moving extremely overweight individuals will cost two and a half times more than what it would cost to transport normal sized people. Several hospitals are outfitting their ambulances with special lift systems to handle the outsize loads.

SUPER CEMETERIES Our nation's cemeteries are getting squeezed more than ever with bigger graves. According to a report in *The New York Times*, the International Cemetery, Cremation and Funeral Association is "worried" that obese corpses can erase upward of four hundred graves in a single-acre plot that would otherwise fit twelve hundred.

SUPER-SIZED THEATER SEATS The average movie seat has increased from twenty inches wide to as much as twenty-six inches; theaters now spend nearly a third more on building space than they did just twenty years ago.

SUPER-SIZED KIDS As of 2017, one in five school children suffers from obesity. When these kids are overweight, they're more likely to develop chronic health conditions—such as asthma and diabetes—and they're more likely to be bullied in school and suffer from depression.

SUPER-SIZED TOILETS Big John, a maker of plus-size toilet seats, provides padded seats that are five inches wider and two inches taller than your standard-issue variety. According to the company's website, the seats can handle upward of twelve hundred pounds.

SUPER-SIZED CLOTHING According to *The Washington Post*, if a size 8 dress from today were sold in 1958, it would actually be considered a size 16.

THE SUPER METABOLISM

This shopping list will provide you with everything you need to harness the full power of your body's energy-burning apparatus:

Super Proteins

- Bison or venison
- Chicken breasts, boneless and skinless
- Eggs
- Fish of all kinds
- Lean beef
- Roast pork
- Turkey
- Whole chicken
- Yogurt

Super Carbs

- Acorn squash
- Amaranth
- Apples
- Bananas
- Barley
- Buckwheat
- Cherries
- Chocolate milk
- Greek yogurt
- Kamut
- Legumes
- Oatmeal
- Potato salad (cold)
- Quinoa
- Sprouted bread
- Sweet potatoes
- Teff

- Triticale
- Wheat bran
- Whole-wheat pasta

Fruits

- All berries
- Apples
- Apricots
- Avocado
- Cherries
- Peaches
- Plums
- Pomegranates

Vegetables

- Artichokes
- Asparagus
- Beans
- Beets
- Bell peppers
- Broccoli
- Brussels sprouts
- Cabbage (all kinds)
- Carrots
- Cauliflower
- Celery
- Cucumbers
- Garlic
- Green beans

TART-UP KIT

- Greens such as spinach, chard, collard, or kale
- Leeks
- Mushrooms
- Onions
- Parsnips
- Peppers
- Radishes
- Rutabagas
- Shallots
- Squash
- Tomatoes
- Turnips

BONUS! Super Snacks

- Any whole fruits (except high-sugar ones)
- Bison jerky
- Carrots
- Deviled eggs
- Fruit salad
- Guacamole
- Hummus
- Kale or other veggie chips

Plus
(See recipes for specific amounts!)

Almond milk
Artichoke hearts
Basil
Chia seeds

Chili powder
Coconut aminos
Cucumber
Curry powder
Dill
Edamame
Fennel
Feta cheese
Ginger
Jalapeño
Lime juice
Mango
Matcha
Milk
Mint
Mussels
Nectarine
Oregano
Organic mayonnaise (such as Wilderness or Spectrum)
Oysters
Parsley
Potatoes
Red pepper flakes
Rice vinegar
Salt and pepper
Seaweed
Shrimp
Tamari
Vanilla extract
Zucchini

Chapter 2

WHY *SUPER METABOLISM?* AND WHY NOW?

Shocking New Scientific Breakthroughs in Nutrition

YOU'RE NOT ALONE in your quest for the body of your dreams. But if you're trying to lose weight on most diets these days, it can certainly feel that way. And usually it all comes down to a single word. Suffice it to say, it's one of my least favorite in the English language.

"No."

We all know the terribly unfulfilling experience of going on a rigorous diet, which is akin to walking through the world like a naked Cersei Lannister in *Game of Thrones*, trailed by a nun shouting, *"Shame!"*

It all begins when you start your day energetically committed to a rigid diet—nibbling at the corners of your food, and practicing restraint as best you possibly can. But before you know it you've transformed yourself into a robotic "no" machine: no to cravings, no to delicious foods, no to exercise (because you're tired), and no to social gatherings. For lunch you said no to the chicken sandwich or cheesy taco and opted instead for a small salad with the dressing on the side. By the time dinnertime rolls around, you've successfully spouted so many no's—and you've deprived yourself of so much food—that you can't help yourself from plundering your kids' unfinished plates of mac and cheese or ordering a pizza from Seamless. What's one drink, you say? Well, have two.

Hey, you'll try again tomorrow.

That's what happens when you're on a quick-fix diet built on a foundation of unrealistic expectations and utter misery: You marble so many no's into your life that you set yourself up to lose in one of life's most enduring forms of self-sabotage. First you lose your confidence, and then if you do succeed in losing weight, you'll lose all over again when you gain it all back—which is sadly the reality for most of us.

According to Kevin Hall, a scientist at the National Institutes of Health, a staggering 80 percent of obese people these days who lose weight dieting will eventually gain it back. That figure gets worse when you understand the consequences: A study published in *The New England Journal of Medicine* last year analyzed data of 9,509 people and found that "yo-yo" dieting may actually double your risk of heart attack or stroke down the road if you suffer from heart disease.

At the end of the day, these diets will all promise you that there is a glorious light at the end of your tunnel: a stellar body. But in the end, it's like what one of my all-time favorite basketball players—the inimitable Charles Barkley—allegedly once said: "Sometimes that light at the end of the tunnel is a train."

Let's be clear: I don't want you to lose. I want you to win.

And that's why I'm loathe to even call the diet enclosed in this book a "diet." I don't believe you should view your weight-loss efforts like an aspiring Navy SEAL who runs up a hill in the middle of the night lugging a log over his shoulders because he wants to pass a test. I don't believe weight loss should ever be so hard. And I refuse to believe that real, meaningful results require suffering.

Forget the log and the hill—the Super Metabolism Diet isn't even a sprint. I would classify it as more of an enduring lifestyle, a way of viewing the world with a greater understanding of your body so you can let it work for you, not *against* you.

Remember, eat *smarter*, not less.

Why You Need to Eat! Eat! Eat!

IF YOU'RE someone who prefers to lose—who enjoys feeling hungry, feeling bloated, and trudging sluggishly through life, let me be very clear: This book is not for you. If you're someone who doesn't enjoy eating tasty, healthy foods and making the easy, necessary changes to improve his or her life, let me be very clear: This book is not for you. And if you're someone who isn't interested in melting excess fat—and looking and feeling amazing with the results—this book is *definitely* not for you. Hey: No judgment here! As a close friend of mine—a successful businessman in New York—likes to say, "Winning isn't for everybody."

But my hunch is that that doesn't apply to you.

Do you know why?

Well, it's because you've already taken one of the biggest and most important steps to winning: You've got a plan. My businessman pal I just mentioned? He'd be the first to tell you that, in business, having a viable plan is the single surefire move that will double your chances of success. The same principle applies to your weight loss. If you don't have a goal in mind, and the right game plan to get there, you're hobbling your chances. So remember:

Super Proteins, Super Carbs, and Super Fats
Up Your Energy Expenditure
Power Snacks
Essential Calories, Vitamins, and Minerals
Relax and Recharge

Now, I'll explain the importance of moving more and upping your energy expenditure in later chapters, but the first step to super-sizing your metabolism is embracing the core pillars of this book:

Super Proteins: Your Metabolic Strongmen (and Lots of Them!)

IF YOUR FOODS were the Avengers, the veggies in your diet are like Captain America. They're wholly good and entirely earnest, like broccoli. Your healthy fats, meanwhile, are slightly more complicated. They're crafty, smart, and sometimes totally irresponsible—not unlike Robert Downey Jr.'s mischievous twist on Iron Man. Your proteins? Without question, they're the mighty Thor, the giant, hammer-wielding god who harnesses the power of thunder and lightning. The guy's all muscle.

You probably already know that eating protein is the key to feeling satisfied with your meals and maintaining any weight-loss effort. Protein is the flubber-frying ingredient for your muscles, and when it comes to burning energy in your body, your muscles are the single most efficient part of your body. On a cellular level, proteins use up way more energy than your more inert fat counterparts—something largely thanks to all of those hardworking, energy-producing mitochondria. Remember that!

More Muscle = More Burn

When you lose muscle mass—whether by aging, lack of exercise, eating the wrong foods, or some combination of the three—your metabolism is guaranteed to get dinged. So feeding your body with plenty of protein is the fundamental building block for building a fully firing metabolism.

Also, simply *eating* protein will burn more calories than if you're eating anything else. As you'll soon learn, a major part of your metabolism is something called the thermic effect of food (TEF), or the energy your body runs through simply digesting what you eat.

Your body works a lot harder to break down those protein molecules into those chains of amino acids than they do other foods. Like meteors trying to enter the earth's atmosphere, much of your protein is burned up on the way in—to the tune of roughly 25 percent. Your carbs and fats, meanwhile, require less work to digest, as only 10 to 15 percent of those get burned up while your body is digesting. Protein is also super satiating and will keep you feeling fuller for much longer, which means you won't be overeating.

Super Proteins—the ones I've selected in this book as the cornerstone of my diet—are simply the best and most efficient foods for building muscle. They also contain all of the essential amino acids, vitamins, and minerals that your body requires.

Now, the Recommended Daily Allowance of protein for men is 56 grams a day, while for women it's 46 grams. That's about as much as you'd get in four to five chicken drumsticks or two large hamburgers. Other ways to reach near those numbers: two and a half pork chops, fifteen slices of bacon, or an 8-ounce steak. But that's *still* not enough: In a 2015 study in the *American Journal of Physiology—Endocrinology and Metabolism,* researchers found that those who ate twice as much protein as the Recommended Daily Allowance had a greater net protein balance and muscle protein synthesis—in other words, it was easier for them to maintain and build muscle, and hence keep their metabolisms revving on high.

In *The Super Metabolism Diet,* I'm recommending you get upwards of 1.6 grams of protein per kilogram of body weight, and even 2 grams per kilogram of body weight if you're working out really hard. If you're a 120-pound woman, you weigh 55 kilograms. That means you'll be eating 88 grams of protein per day. That translates to (roughly):

- Three eggs (23 grams)
- Greek yogurt (one serving = 20 grams)
- Chicken breast (6 ounces = 40 grams)

Upping your protein isn't just an athlete's strategy for bulking up—it's also the best way for all of us to slim down. After all, what do Rocky Balboa and Kim Kardashian have in common? They both rely on plenty of protein to get their bodies in tip-top shape. While Rocky chugged raw eggs before his a.m. runs, Kim K. revealed that she sneaks protein into each of her meals and snacks to get back to her pre-baby weight.

While the stars may each have vastly different goals—Rocky's goal to kick butt in the boxing ring, Kim's goal to slay in couture evening wear—they're both smart to make protein a cornerstone of their diets. The nutrient fuels the muscle-building process, dulls hunger, and can help prevent obesity, diabetes, and heart disease! And while most of us know about at least some of these benefits, few of us are eating the proper amount.

If that's not enough to sell you on a high-protein diet, remember that it . . .

● Builds new tissues in your body.
● Helps you digest your food (as enzymes).
● Transports oxygen throughout your body.

It doesn't hurt that your favorite proteins taste pretty darn good, too.

Super Fats: Your Crafty Frenemies

IT'S EASY TO view fats as villainous. Yes, it's the same stuff that accumulates around your belly. It's likely the reason you're holding this book. And yes, fats were the food-world bogeyman for pretty much the whole of the twentieth century. But it's a different world now: Today people carry high-powered computers in their pockets, Pluto is no longer a planet, and the Cubs are officially the World Series champs.

Also, we've learned that our bodies simply require dietary fat (which is why many fats are called "essential") in order to lose weight and function properly. The right kinds of fats help increase satiety, maximize your metabolism, protect against heart disease, speed nutrients through your body, and improve your fat-soluble vitamin uptake. Not to mention, most unprocessed, high-fat foods also come jam-packed with many of those important nutrients, from vitamins and minerals to free-radical-fighting antioxidants.

The fact that many Americans still haven't shaken off the decades-long notion that fat—and particularly saturated fat—is bad for you isn't even the biggest issue we face in adopting more fats into our diets. Many of us struggle to determine which fats we should be eating because the US Dietary Guidelines (and nutrition labels) are both generalizing and misleading. According to the guidelines, reducing saturated fat could lower the risk of heart disease if those fats are replaced with a type of "good fat" known as polyunsaturated fat. The only problem is that both heart-healthy omega-3s and inflammation-inducing, fat-storing omega-6s are included in that type of fat, and most Americans are already getting twenty times the amount of omega-6s we really need, according to an analysis by researchers at the University of Maryland Medical Center.

The reality is, not all fats are created equal. Some are downright bad, some are misunderstood, and some fats are, well, flat-out Super. And, don't get me wrong, eating foods that are packed with the wrong kinds of fat *will* make you fat, but with all the omegas, and monos, and polys out there, it can be kind of confusing which are which.

Here's the quick skinny on fats.

The Good (a.k.a.: Super Fats)

THESE ARE minimally processed to nonprocessed foods that are full of unsaturated fats, heart-healthy, polyunsaturated omega-3 fatty acids (ALA, DHA, and EPA), monounsaturated fats (OEA [oleic acid]), and the single trans fat conjugated linoleic acid (CLA), as well as some medium-chain saturated fats like stearic acid and lauric acid. These are also the fats found in nature, from glorious foods like avocado, nuts, eggs, certain fish, and healthy oils such as olive oil. This is the healthy fat that helps you control your weight and strengthen your heart. And get this: They also help you burn fat—especially the monosaturated fats, which are the ones contained in nuts, avocados, and olives. Here are the best of the best:

Lauric Acid

Sources: Coconut oil, palm kernel oil (not to be confused with palm oil)

What it does: The body doesn't convert medium-chain saturated fatty acids, also known as medium-chain triglycerides, into body fat as easily as it does other types of dietary fat. That means it's less likely to be stored in your body and more likely to be burned for energy. Lauric acid acts as an antimicrobial when used externally, which means a slathering of coconut oil can help stave off infections by killing bacteria. And while lauric acid does increase total cholesterol levels more than many other fatty acids, most of this rise is because of the increase in high-density lipoprotein (HDL), the "good" cholesterol.

Stearic Acid

Sources: Cocoa butter, shea butter, grass-fed beef, milk, and butter

What it does: Stearic acid is a type of long-chain saturated fat, whose long length contributes to its digestion-slowing properties—which can help flatten your belly by keeping you fuller longer. It plays a key role in regulating the performance of mitochondria, the energy-producing powerhouses of our cells. And in clinical studies, stearic acid was found to be associated with lowered LDL cholesterol and inflammation in comparison to other saturated fats. As for where you can get stearic acid on the reg? Grass-fed beef is higher in stearic acid and lower in unhealthy palmitic acid than conventionally raised beef, and dark chocolate that's higher than 70 percent cacao has the most stearic-acid-containing cocoa butter.

Omega-9s

Sources: Olive oil, avocados, walnuts, canola oil, peanut oil, macadamia nuts

What it does: Oleic acid (OEA), also known as omega-9, is the primary monounsaturated fat found in olive oil, but it's also found in sunflower oil, grapeseed oil, and sesame oil. Oleic acid can help reduce appetite and promote weight loss. Studies have shown that a higher intake of monounsaturated fat may raise the "good" high-density lipoprotein (HDL) cholesterol without raising the "bad" low-density lipoprotein (LDL) cholesterol. It's also been found to enhance uptake of essential fat-burning nutrients compared to other oils while down-regulating expression of certain fat genes. Additionally, research out of the University of California, Irvine, found that this particular type of fat boosts memory.

Omega-3s

Eicosapentaenoic acid (EPA) and docosahexaenoic acid (DHA)

Sources: Fish, algae supplements like spirulina

What it does: EPA and DHA are the sea-based versions of omega-3s. Research shows that they are more active in the body than ALA (the plant-based version) at controlling inflammation and belly fat. A report in the journal *Nutrition in Clinical Practice* found that these omega-3s decrease the production of cytokines—inflammation-promoting compounds produced by harmful belly fat—and improve fat metabolism by altering the expression of inflammatory genes. Not only that, but other studies connect their intake with a reduced risk of heart disease and Alzheimer's. DHA, in particular, has been found to be essential in the growth and development of infants' brains as well as for normal brain function in adults. To get some extra DHA in your diet, pick up sardines, sockeye salmon, rainbow trout, or canned light tuna.

Alpha-linoleic acid (ALA)

Sources: Flaxseeds, chia seeds, walnuts, kiwi, hemp, canola oil, grass-fed beef

What it does: ALA is an omega-3 and an essential fatty acid, meaning it cannot be produced by the body. Like all omega-3s, it helps to reduce appetite, control inflammation, and promote weight loss, and studies specific to ALA have found that it plays a role in reducing the risk of heart attacks, lowering cholesterol levels as well as blood pressure. But because our body has to convert ALA into the active forms of EPA and, more importantly, DHA before it can be used, some researchers suggest you'd have to increase your intake of ALAs to get a benefit equal to the fish-based sources. A surprising bonus, grass-fed beef is higher in omega-3s than their conventionally raised counterparts because grass contains higher levels of ALA than corn or soy.

Arachidonic acid

Sources: Duck, chicken, halibut, wild salmon, eggs (yolks), beef

What it does: Like EPA and DHA, arachidonic acid (AA or ARA) is a precursor that is metabolized into a wide range of biologically important acids. Supplementation of AA has been shown to increase lean body mass, strength, and anaerobic power in men. In a study at the University of Tampa, men who took ARA gained 1.62 kilograms of lean muscle mass versus 0.09 for those who took a placebo. ARA also accounts for 10 percent of the brain's fat content.

Conjugated Linoleic acid

Sources: Grass-fed beef and grass-fed dairy, turkey, lamb, veal

What it does: Naturally occurring trans fats, like conjugated linoleic acids (CLA), are produced in the guts of cows, turkeys, and lamb (but not chickens or pigs) and hence the foods made from these animals (e.g., milk products and meat). A review of eighteen studies of human subjects in *The American Journal of Clinical Nutrition* found that CLA produces modest reductions in body fat in humans. It's also a powerful antioxidant, and may be protective against heart disease, cancer, and diabetes. Grass-fed beef contains an average of two to three times more CLA than grain-fed beef.

The Complicated

SATURATED FATTY ACIDS are composed of chains that are made up of only single bonds. Because this orientation is ordered and relatively straight, it is easy for these kinds of fats to pack together tightly, which is a reason why saturated fats—butters, the fats in red meats, and coconut oil—are solid at room temperature. Many studies, including a comprehensive meta-analysis in the *Annals of Internal Medicine,* have concluded that there is no significant evidence that saturated fat increases your risks for cardiovascular diseases, and consuming the right types of saturated fat in moderation can actually help you torch body fat. Some of the best examples are lean beef and coconut.

The Downright Evil

YOU'VE PROBABLY heard of trans fats. These are the nasty creations that are loaded in everything from your candy bars to the gooey, heart-stopping mess that someone pours on your movie-theater popcorn.

When I say "creation," I mean it. Trans fats are the Frankenstein's monster of the food world—fully human inventions that are wholly unnatural: They include margarine, fried and battered foods, doughnuts (or any baked goods that are produced on a mass scale), and frozen pizzas. Trans fats do two things really, really effectively: They up your low-density lipoprotein (LDL), the bad cholesterol that clogs your arteries, while reducing your high-density lipoprotein (HDL), the good stuff that helps your body process any of that extra cholesterol. All of this increases your risk of type 2 diabetes, heart attack, and stroke.

When your heart isn't pumping as much blood, you're not circulating as much oxygen to your cells, which means your all-important metabolism isn't firing at full force.

Here are some of the worst of the worst:

Partially hydrogenated oils

Sources: Fried foods, baked goods, shortening/margarine

What it does: Several decades ago, scientists discovered that if they injected vegetable oil with hydrogen via "partially hydrogenating" the oil, it would turn solid—and stay that way, even at room temperature. Unfortunately, these unconjugated trans fatty acids (which are primarily made up of a fat called elaidic acid) also tend to turn solid once they're inside your body, where they jam up your arteries, including those in your brain. This man-made fat is now banned by the Food and Drug Administration (FDA) because it's been shown to increase the risk of heart disease (by increasing LDL and decreasing HDL), weight gain, and stroke while diminishing memory—making it one of the worst foods for your brain.

Vaccenic acid

Sources: Grass-fed beef and grass-fed dairy, turkey, lamb, veal

What it does: Even though this type of trans fat is naturally occurring, it may be just as bad as the industrial fats—which is why manufacturers have to include it on their Nutrition Facts Panel under "Trans Fats" alongside the fake stuff. (Interestingly, the "good" trans fat, CLA, is not included because it does not fit the FDA's definition of a trans fat.) According to a study published in *The American Journal of Clinical Nutrition,* both industrial trans fats and vaccenic acid (VA) increase LDL cholesterol. However, it isn't all bad news; VA also moderately increases HDL cholesterol, whereas industrial trans fats do not. Although this natural trans fat may not be the best for your health in equal amounts to industrial trans fats, luckily, we don't consume as much of it. Industrial trans fats can make up to 9 percent of our total energy intake whereas these naturally occurring trans fats rarely exceed 0.5 percent, according to a review in *Nature Reviews Endocrinology.*

Linoleic acid

Sources: Soybean oil, safflower oil, corn oil, poppy seed oil

What it does: An omega-6 fatty acid, linoleic acid accounts for 85 to 90 percent of the omega-6 fatty acids in our diet. In a review in the journal *Nutrition,* researchers reported that linoleic acid has been shown to be possibly adipogenic, which means it promotes fat storage in our bodies. On the other hand, the omega-3, alpha-linolenic acid (ALA), may promote lipid oxidation.

Palmitic acid

Sources: Palm oil, conventionally raised animal fats

What it does: Excess carbohydrates in the body are converted into palmitic acid. As a result, it is a major body component of animals, but even more so in conventionally raised, grain-fed animals than in grass-fed animals. Palmitic acid may increase your risk of heart disease due to its effect on cholesterol levels: A meta-analysis in *The Journal of Nutrition* found that palm oil significantly increases low-density lipoprotein (LDL), or bad cholesterol, compared with vegetable oils low in saturated fat. On top of that, a separate study found that rats fed a diet of palmitic acid and carbs showed a suppression of the body's signaling from leptin and insulin, the key hormones involved in weight regulation and appetite suppression.

At the end of the day, you've got to eat fat to lose fat—but only the good kind. Also, when you do so, you'll slow the sugar into your bloodstream so your blood-sugar levels are more stable and your metabolism can keep humming.

Super Carbs: Your Essential Wingmen

YES, ADVISING YOU to boost your carb intake will sound like heresy to all of the hard-core fitness buffs of the world who desperately cling to the notion that all carbs are evil. And to their credit, some carbs are fairly close to evil. They're called refined carbohydrates—the fiber-less stuff found in sweets and white bread, pasta, flour, etc.—and they're one of the prime supervillains who will wreak havoc on your blood-sugar levels and ultimately your metabolism as a whole. (For more on that, read on.) But carbs aren't just defined by the nutrient-less stuff you find in Wonder Bread. Complex carbs from whole grains and veggies are necessary for good health and a flat belly.

Remember the old children's story *Goldilocks and the Three Bears*? Little Goldilocks found that the bears' porridge was either too hot, too cold, or just right.

When it comes to carbs, Super Carbs are the ones that are "just right." They're found in whole foods that come jam-packed with vital nutrients, and they fall in a necessary sweet spot: They provide your metabolism with essential sugars to burn and also come packed with enough fiber to ensure that our blood-sugar levels don't spiral out of control. And as you'll soon learn, you'll be better off ingesting your favorite carbs at night.

Combine a diet based on those pillars with various high-protein Super Snacks to keep your body burning and your metabolism humming, and other super strategies (which you'll learn about later), and you're guaranteed to start shedding pounds and feeling better than you've ever felt before.

If you keep eating the wrong foods, you won't like what happens. Trust me.

Why Calorie Counting Doesn't Work

WE LIVE IN a data-driven world.

Chances are you walk through life with a smartphone tracking your every move from the moment you wake up until the moment you crawl into bed at night after a long day. In 2018, everything from healthcare to fighting crime has become a game of numbers. Right now, thanks to data, the folks at Google are always working to pinpoint an exact profile for who you are so they can predict how you like to shop so they can serve you the most effective advertisements possible. (Facebook, meanwhile, knows exactly who you are, because you've told them.) In the baseball world, "sabremetrics" wizards can tell you which first baseman in a Major League Baseball team's farm system has the highest probability of advancing a runner with a base hit in a two-out situation. Heck, there are data whizzes who are fans of TV's dating show *The Bachelor* who can tell you that, on average, the typical bachelor opts for a winner who is six years younger than he is, and the typical bachelorette tends to go for a man exactly one year older than she is.

Given the obesity epidemic in the United States, you'd think that the world of weight loss might have a better data-based model by now. But the reality is that we don't, and far too many people still cling to the wildly outdated—but still tantalizingly simple—model of "calories in, calories out."

KNOW THY SUGARS

NOT ALL SUGARS ARE CREATED EQUAL. HERE ARE THE THREE WAYS YOU EXERCISE YOUR SWEET TOOTH.

Sucrose: This is also known as basic table sugar, the crystallized stuff that someone harvested from a sugarcane plant. You'll find it like snow atop doughnuts, in large bottles at the diner for pouring into your coffee mug, and in recipes for your favorite sweets. Its molecules are composed of half glucose, half fructose, and it splits into those inside your body.

Glucose: This is the sugar your body uses to fuel your metabolism and is burned off in your cells as energy.

Fructose: This is the sugar that you'll find in nature, typically fruits and honey. You'll also find it in high-fructose corn syrup, soft drinks, and sugar substitutes. When consumed in whole fruits, it's accompanied by fiber, and your body handles the fructose load easily—like Derek Jeter fielding a routine grounder. When you eat too much fructose, however, terrible things happen. In addition to increasing blood pressure and heart rate, it wreaks havoc on your liver, which can't handle it all, before it's stored as triglycerides—or fats. That's like Jeter trying to handle eighty-seven grounders at once.

It's understandable, of course. When you're talking about your metabolism, it's easy to simplify everything to a string of numbers.

After all, as you'll learn from this book, it's an equation!

Let's say you've calculated your total energy expenditure to roughly 2,400 calories a day. Again, that's what you need for everything—the energy you need to function, digest your food, move around, and even exercise. Then, the thinking goes, if you eat 2,400 calories on the nose, you won't gain a single pound. Let's set aside the whole notion that all calories aren't created equal. Now, by that measure, you can, in theory, subtract 400 or 500 calories from your diet and achieve what scientists call a "negative energy balance." In normal terms, that means the pounds will simply melt off. Or, as the mean, overly dramatic cheerleader coach in the classic teen movie *Bring It On* explained to his exhausted pupils as they trained for their big competition: "I want you to think of what you ate today. Got it? Now, cut that in half! This is called a diet, people!"

Though I appreciate the enthusiasm, I'm instantly reminded of Einstein's famous—if apocryphal—quote: "Everything should be made as simple as possible, but not simpler." In other words, just because his explanation is wonderfully understandable doesn't mean it's actually correct. In fact, the coach's flat-out wrong.

First off, you can reach 2,400 calories in Snickers bars and movie-theater popcorn just as easily as you can whole foods and protein shakes. But even if you're eating great, nutritious foods, cutting calories is the equivalent of taking a monkey wrench to your metabolism's knees.

If you recall, in the introduction to this book I mentioned a study that focused in on the weight-loss efforts of contestants of NBC's wildly popular series *The Biggest Loser*, the show in which overweight or obese people suffer through harsh eating and fitness regimens as they compete for prizes based on the amount of weight they lose.

The study, conducted by researchers at the National Institutes of Health, and published in 2016 in the journal *Obesity*, tracked the weights and hormones of sixteen contestants, some of whom had lost literally hundreds of pounds. One guy, named Danny Cahill, managed to shed 239 pounds over the course of seven months! According to Withings, the digital scale manufacturer, Cahill lost the equivalent of thirty-six billion grains of sand—or roughly the same weight as 191 leather basketballs piled on top of one another.

The extreme weight loss came with consequences.

When the show started, the contestants had metabolisms on par for someone their original sizes. By the end, their metabolisms were severely hobbled and weren't fast enough even to power their smaller frames. Most disconcerting was the fact that their metabolisms never actually came back to full power. Mr. Cahill, in fact, regained more than one hundred pounds.

What happened inside their suffering bodies?

Well, it was a number of factors, but a chief reason, according to the researchers, was the influence of leptin, the body's hormone that tells you that you're satiated, or no longer hungry. Over the course of the crash diet, the contestant's leptin levels essentially flatlined and then never fully came back. The researchers also targeted their ghrelin levels—the hormone that tells you when you're hungry—which had actually risen.

In effect, they reprogrammed their bodies to be fat-storing, low-energy machines.

Torture Yourself—and Pay the Consequences

NOW, YOU DON'T have to be going to the extremes of *The Biggest Loser* contestants to achieve the same feat. The stories are legion.

For a study published in *The American Journal of Clinical Nutrition,* in 2015, researchers from Germany's University of Kiel took thirty-two non-obese males and slashed their calories by an average of 1,300 for simply a *three-wee*k period. On the whole, the subjects emerged having gained weight while seeing a dramatic decrease in muscle mass—roughly 5 percent across the board. Their leptin levels plummeted by 44 percent.

By the end, the total number of calories they were burning per day had slowed by 266.

In a study of rats published in the February 2017 issue of *Physiological*

SUPER METABOLISM BOOST!

Small change, big results!

HOLSTER YOUR PHONE!

Reason number 3,485 you should unplug during part of your days: Researchers at the National Institute on Drug Abuse have found that just fifty minutes of cellphone use a day can affect your brain's glucose metabolism—or its ability to burn energy!

Reports, researchers from Kent State University cut their calories by 50 percent over a three-week period only to see their resting energy expenditure decline by 40 percent and their non-resting energy expenditure decline by 48 percent.

At the end of the day, treating yourself like a lab rat and putting yourself through the agony of a harsh negative energy balance can have disastrous consequences on even more than your metabolism.

It's one of the most important pillars of a Super Metabolism: You need to be eating *enough* foods and not starving yourself to keep your body operating at peak capacity.

A DEAR JOHN LETTER TO YOUR JUICER

Breaking up is always hard to do. But if you want a fully charged, fully optimized metabolism, it's time to let one of your all-time favorite kitchen appliances go—once and for all.

Dear Beloved Electric Juice Master X-955,

There's no easy way to do this, so I'm just going to come out and say it. It's over.

I'm sorry, I really am. It's not you, it's me. Actually, it's a little bit both of us. It's about the way you put things into me. It's complicated.

You're beautiful. You really are. I truly believe that you're an amazing vessel for pulverizing food and ensuring that I get a lot of fruits and vegetables in easy and tasty ways. And that's what makes this whole breakup thing really, really hard.

Before you say anything, no, this isn't about the time I almost left you for a Cuisinart Juicer. This is something different. I'm not falling for the next flashy young thing that promises digestive miracles. I'm rethinking my whole relationship with food, and I realize that you're not so great for me or my metabolism.

I don't know if you read a lot of nutritional research—do juicers keep up on that kind of thing?—but there was a study published earlier this year in the *Journal of the American College of Cardiology* that gave me pause. They found that the process of juicing fruits or vegetables "concentrates calories, which makes it much easier to ingest too many." Remember that delicious juice we made together yesterday, which had spinach and berries and apples and yogurt and walnuts? It's like 500 calories. No, seriously. I looked it up! That's just a little less than a Big Mac.

That'd be okay if I stopped with one. But I drank that smoothie in twenty seconds and thought, "Mmm, that was tasty and yummy. I should have another." And you totally helped me do it! You were like, "Sure, make another. Put some peanut butter in it this time. It's all healthy!" There's no nice way to say it, man. You're an enabler.

This isn't just me whining. It's been proven with science. Drinking doesn't satiate like chewing food, so by creating a meal with you my caloric intake could increase by 15 percent every day. Chewing exists for a reason. It helps monitor how much I'm eating. But with a juice or smoothie, thanks to yours truly, I don't have that "crunch effect" anymore. It's all slurping. A slurp doesn't resonate like a crunch. A slurp doesn't say, "You know, if you keep going down this road, we're gonna end up wearing sweatpants to work, right?"

I know that you have the best of intentions. You're trying to help me make better dietary choices. But you're just a juicer, so you can't be expected to understand the complexities of the human digestive system. In your limited metallic brain, you think, "I made him eat a bunch of fruits and vegetables. He must be super-healthy now!"

But it's not that simple.

It's also because you took out the fiber. Not all the fiber, mind you. You left me with the soluble fiber, which is easily absorbed by water. But when you hack it up with your well-meaning blades, you take out the insoluble fiber, which is sometimes known as the roughage. It's the stalks, skins, and seeds. It's not good for drinking, but when it gets into my body, it limits how much sugar is absorbed by my liver. If I bite into an apple, those two fibers— the soluble and insoluble—work together to make sure my body isn't being overwhelmed. The soluble fiber is like, "You want some sugar? Let's get this party started!" But the insoluble fiber is like, "Whoa, whoa, whoa, let's slow it down. You'll get your sugar. But first, how about some nutrients? You scratch our back, we'll scratch yours."

I'm sorry, juicer, but it's over. I want my mouth to communicate responsibly about hunger with my brain, based on chewing, digestion, and not on speed. I don't want my liver to get blitzkrieged by sugar just because I don't want to use a fork. I don't want to get tricked into thinking a wheelbarrow full of food is okay to eat just because I can shotgun it. We've had some good times you and I, juicer, but I can't do this anymore. It's starting to feel abusive. So I'm ending it. It's for my metabolism. If I'm looking for some juice these days, I'm going to opt for a good old blender. When you blend fruits and vegetables, the resulting liquids contains all of the good stuff I need. In fact, a study by food scientists at Texas A&M University actually proved it. Juices that were blended had way higher levels of fiber and beneficial phytonutrients—and seven times more naringin, an anti-inflammatory phytochemical that may help fight cancer— compared to the stuff created by your cousin, Mr. Electric Juicer.

So leave the blueberries and apples slices where you found them.

Don't call me. I'll call you.

Chapter 3

BURN FAT DAY AND NIGHT

How Your Superpower Shapes Your Body— and How It Can Change It

YOUR PARENTS TOLD you to do this. So did your kindergarten teacher. Even self-help spoofer Stuart Smalley on *Saturday Night Live*. Now, it's my turn. If you can, find a nearby mirror and look deeply into your own eyes. Take a large gulp of air and exhale slowly. Find your "center," as the yogis say. Then repeat after me: "You're special."

I'll admit: It's a little corny. And yes, I know this sort of earnest self-helpness has fallen out of favor in today's day and age, when leading psychologists and tough-loving parents believe the whole "everyone deserves a trophy"-type thinking is a recipe for narcissism and failure. But whether or not that's true, I'm not your shrink, and I'm not asking you to perform this exercise for your ego or your sense of mental well-being. (Which, let's be clear, I hope is strong.) I'm telling you this because knowing your true and inherent uniqueness will set you on the path to unlocking your body's secrets and help you finally take control of your life in ways that you've never even imagined.

Here's the thing: You *are* special. You're like a snowflake. As part of our species, you may be a single droplet in an ocean of seven billion humans who have evolved over the last two hundred thousand years, but there are certain characteristics that you and only you have. You've got your own fingerprints, your own genome, your own personality. In recent years, researchers have found that you may even have your own signature ways of thinking and viewing the world. In a recent study published in the journal *Nature Neuroscience*, researchers from Yale University, using images from functional magnetic resonance imaging (fMRI) brain scans, found evidence that we each have a unique neurological "fingerprint" within our neural networks. Meanwhile, in Japan, researchers at Osaka University created software that can identify individuals in a crowd with up to 95 percent accuracy by simply analyzing their gaits. In other words, congrats! You have your own signature stroll.

The same goes for your metabolism.

Your Metabolism Is Unique

IF YOU'RE GOING to unleash the full power of your metabolism—and burn all that extra fat and finally get the body of your dreams—it's important to understand that metabolism is something that also varies from person to person. After all, who doesn't have that one friend who lives his or her life like some genetically enhanced mutant in an *X-Men* movie, capable of wolfing down a dozen Dunkin' Donuts—or tall, wobbly stacks of Five Guys cheeseburgers—and yet somehow manages to lose weight? These freakish overeaters among us have diets that would make any nutritionist worth his or her salt cringe, yet they walk through life lean, happy, and carefree.

Yes, they're annoying. And I'll be the first to admit that it's easy to feel discouraged, eye them with envy, and ultimately write yourself off as some loser in the great genetic lottery.

To date, conventional medicine has no viable explanation for why some people can devour certain foods and vaporize the calories while others can't. "Precision medicine recognizes that we each have a distinct metabolic makeup," says Florence Comite, MD, a respected New York–based endocrinologist and leader in the field of precision medicine. "And metabolism is very dynamic."

If your metabolism is sluggish, genetics may indeed be playing a role. What works for someone else may not work for you, and vice versa. "Somebody from a certain genetic background, cultural, or even ethnic background—the way they eat and the way they metabolize can be completely different than someone from a different one," says UT Southwestern's Dr. Mangelsdorf. "Northern Europeans have a completely different metabolic phenotype than people that are native from Africa, or India, or Native Americans."

Amazing, right?

But that doesn't mean you can't take control with the key, universal lifestyle choices contained in this book that are specifically designed to optimize your superpower and getting it firing at full force.

At the end of the day, the metabolic hand you're dealt is only the beginning, not the end. That means you shouldn't fold and trust in the fate of the genetic gods. Trust me: You're firmly in control. It's time to start making some small and easy, fundamental changes to your diet—and embracing the movement plan contained in this book—that will get your metabolism online.

Fourteen days.

That's all I'm asking for. It may sound like a long time. And, in some respects, it is (especially if—like many Americans—that's the stretch between two paychecks). But believe me, you'll be shocked at how easy it is to stick to this plan with only the slightest commitment. Remember: You're the hero!

During those two weeks you'll put a stop to all of the harmful habits you're engaged in on a daily basis that negatively impact your superpower, and by the time you reach day fifteen, you'll have the tools you need—and a truly supercharged metabolism—to carry you for the rest of your life.

However, before you embark on your quest to uncover your inner strength and start living your life with more energy and a more positive spirit than ever, you need to know what constitutes your superpower in the first place.

The Factory Inside You

IF YOU HAPPENED to cruise the floor of a medical conference cluttered with the world's foremost physicians, endocrinologists, and dieticians, and you asked twenty different individuals for the definition of "metabolism," there's a good chance you'd get twenty different answers. For a word we casually fling around with such regularity—"yeah, my friend Samantha has a *totally fast* metabolism"—it never ceases to amaze me how few of us can actually define it. (Dinner party trick: Challenge your friends to "define the word 'metabolism' in one sentence.") That's because the metabolic process is so wildly complex, and it involves basically the whole of the human body—literally trillions upon trillions of cells.

Honestly, you'd be better off going to Comic-Con and asking a *Star Wars* buff to give you a working definition of "The Force."

"In my class, for example, in defining metabolism, I always show my students a composite definition culled from Dictionary .com, Merriam-Webster, and the Cambridge dictionary," says

Clyde Wilson, PhD, an instructor at Stanford University, a research associate at the University of California, San Francisco, and director of the Center for Nutrition at the Sports Medicine Institute—who also happens to be one of the world's foremost experts on the science of metabolism. "And then we [try to pin down] a functionally relevant version of the definition from there."

Generally speaking, your metabolism is defined as all of the biochemical reactions that take place inside every single cell of your body—or any body, for that matter—to keep you alive. After all, every living organism needs some form of metabolism to survive, including plants. (Remember photosynthesis from third-grade science? That's half of a plant's metabolism. The other half is respiration, or the release of carbon dioxide.) Here's a fun fact: Hummingbirds, with their tiny bodies and their rapid-fire, machine-gun wings, have the fastest metabolisms on the planet. They're such little burning cauldrons, they have to woof down their entire body weight in food every single day just to maintain their body temperature. The animal with the slowest metabolism on record? That's the glacially slow-moving three-toed sloth, native to Central and South America, which needs astonishingly little energy—only 162 kilojoules per day per kilogram of body weight (which, in food terms, translates to fewer calories than you'd find in a single bite of an apple)—to survive.

Your metabolism, meanwhile, falls somewhere in between. It operates based on a host of factors and ultimately boils down to a process in your cells that allows your body to take the substrates

SUPER METABOLISM BOOST!

Small change, big results!

KEEP COOL

Heat up your fuel burning by keeping things cool at home. Research published in *The Journal of Clinical Investigation* reveals that exposure to temperatures between 60 and 61 degrees Fahrenheit over a ten-day period saw significant increases in healthy brown adipose tissue, the kind that can increase metabolism and burn dangerous visceral fat.

from your food—from the protein, sugar, and fat molecules you digest—and either store them away in your body or release them as energy.

Your body, however, isn't a simple, mouth-to-cells plumbing network. There are several things that influence your metabolism and how well it does its job. Physical activity plays a part. So do sleep quality and your stress levels. Heck, just as you learned on the previous page, even the temperature in your home can play a role in your body's energy-releasing apparatus.

Your hormones, meanwhile, are absolutely critical to your metabolic machinery, especially insulin, cortisol, testosterone, human growth hormone, and your thyroid hormones. (After all, as you'll soon learn, your thyroid gland is your body's inner metabolic conductor.) But the foundation of your metabolism, of course, is your diet.

Without your metabolism, your body wouldn't be able to sustain itself and perform everyday physiological things you never even think about, such as circulating blood, digesting food, breathing, dividing your cells, and healing. In fact, scientists have estimated that roughly 60 to 80 percent of all the energy your body produces goes to simply staying alive and keeping your body humming.

Think about that. The vast majority of *all* the energy you burn isn't for moving around, cycling to work, hitting the gym, or playing with your kids. It goes to basic bodily functions, such as digesting your food, beating your heart, and, well, *thinking.* Your metabolism is burning up tiny bits of energy right now to keep your eyes—and your occipital lobe, the part of the brain that processes printed words—focused on this page. As I stated previously, your noggin, though only roughly 2 percent of your body weight, is responsible for upward of 20 percent of your total energy expenditure! Reading books, taking standardized tests, gazing at sunsets, and cleansing itself of toxins while you're snoring in bed—science hasn't a clue where all of those calories are going inside your neural framework, specifically—but it's generally understood that running your physiology is difficult business, and your brain is essentially a very demanding machine that hoovers up a ton of calories.

So, if you ever needed a reminder about the importance of eating right, remember that fact: The vast majority of calories you consume go *directly* to keeping your body's factory humming along as usual—not for fueling exercise. The name for your base-level metabolism, simply to function? It's called your basal metabolic rate (BMR). Combine that with the energy you need to move around physically (roughly 20 percent of your energy use) and what's called the thermic effect of food (TEF)—which is the energy you need to digest food, or 5 to 10 percent of your energy use—and you've got your metabolism, also known as your total energy expenditure (TEE).

Now, if you Google "metabolism," you're bound to discover millions of articles that describe it as the "engine" of your body. You know: You're the car and your food is the fuel, and your metabolism is the internal combustion engine that converts all of those eggs, sandwiches, and steak dinners into white-hot energy that powers your body. While I appreciate the simplicity of the metaphor, I think we can do better. A lot better.

Your body is more like a factory.

Your body is a sprawling and complex organization with near-countless departments working together—which include your hormones, your organs, your enzymes, even your immune system—which, if jibing in perfect harmony, are churning out a product called energy and storing away a product called fat. Sometimes there's miscommunication among your departments, and a lot of outside factors influence your factory. Your factory can't run all the time. It needs to power down properly at night for cleaning to be fresh in the morning. If an accident occurs and creates stress, your whole system gets disrupted.

And when you cut staff in any of the departments—or find that some are underperforming—the factory as a whole suffers, and less energy gets burned, and more and more fat gets piled high like the stacks and stacks of pallets you'll see in any major corporate warehouse.

Now, if your average fitness model has a body like an Amazon .com warehouse—where super cool, high-tech robots dart across the floors and swiftly complete tasks with laser-like precision—your own body could be more like some ancient widget maker. You're overpaying the wrong people, your outdated communication system is a mess, your employee morale is in the cellar, and you're churning a fraction of the energy that you should be producing. So consider this book your own personal private equity wiz, here to show you how to be a leaner, better, smarter, and more efficient operation.

Remember: Eat *smarter*, not less.

And it all begins with calling HR—human resources—and sitting down the worst parts of your diet—the raw materials you're bringing into it to create energy—and telling it, point-blank: "You're fired."

Then you'll reward the right players in your metabolic machine with the bonuses and staff up elsewhere. In no time, your efficiency will rise.

ENERGY DEPENDENCE: WHERE DOES IT ALL GO?
A BRIEF GLOSSARY OF OFFICIAL (A.K.A. "SUPER WONKY!") METABOLISM TERMINOLOGY

BASAL METABOLIC RATE (BMR) OR RESTING METABOLIC RATE (RMR): This one's easy to remember. Basal? It may sound like something related to your nose, but it's actually just another way of saying "base layer," and this refers to all of the calories you burn when you're doing, well, nothing—when you're lying down and taking a nap, reading a book, sitting through a painstakingly boring meeting at your office, or watching episodes 22 through 37 of *House of Cards* in a single weekend. Think of it as your base-layer metabolism. Between 60 and 80 percent of all of your daily calories go to you BMR. This encompasses all of the energy you need for basic physiological processes such as heartbeat and, well, consciousness.

THERMIC EFFECT OF FOOD (TEF): As I mentioned before: Just like a meteor that falls from the heavens and gets burned up entering the earth's atmosphere, your food gets broken down as it travels through your digestive tract. And this term refers to all of the calories your body burns simply to digest your food. It represents anywhere from 10 to 30 percent of the calories you consume.

NON-EXERCISE ACTIVITY THERMOGENESIS (NEAT): As the title suggests, this is the term for energy burn that isn't exercise but is still considered "activity." If you're someone who walks a lot but doesn't hit the gym, you'll be plenty NEAT. That's because it's the term for all of the energy your body burns for everything we do except sleeping, eating, or physical exercise. In other words, it includes fidgeting, standing, painting, and typing on your computer. It's responsible for anywhere between 15 and 20 percent of your metabolism.

EXCESS POST-EXERCISE OXYGEN CONSUMPTION (EPOC): Have you ever done something physically rigorous, and your body continues to feel hot afterward? Your heart rate is up, your skin feels like a stovetop to the touch, and your body keeps sweating long after you've toweled off following your post-exercise shower?

Well, your body continues to burn energy after performing a workout as it works to bring your body back to normal. (To borrow a metaphor from the American Council on Exercise, it's like an engine that remains hot after a long drive.) It can mean anywhere from an extra 50 to 200 calories burned following a hard workout.

EXERCISE (EX): Yes, that. Roughly 20 percent of your calorie burn comes from moving your muscles.

TOTAL ENERGY EXPENDITURE (TEE): The overarching term for your "metabolism." Meaning: all of the above combined. If you want to get all algebraic with it, it's calculated using this basic formula:

$$TEE = RMR + TEF + NEAT + EPOC + EX$$

"I'LL SHOW YOU MY RATE IF YOU SHOW ME YOURS."

The secrets for calculating your metabolism at home

THERE'S SO much stuff I wish I could tell you. Did Tony Soprano die in the final episode of *The Sopranos,* or did he happily finish off that plate of onion rings and simply go home? Did we *really* walk on the moon? Who was Jack the Ripper? How much did Tom Brady *really* know about Deflategate?

On top of that long list, I would add, simply: "your metabolism."

Seriously. I wish that I was indeed some sort of metabolism whisperer who could look you directly in the eye and say, "Janice, your TEE is 2,100 calories. That's what you burn every day."

But, as I mentioned earlier, I don't have that power. But, guess what? You do! (Remember, *you're* the hero of this journey—I'm merely your guide.)

If you really wish to pinpoint your metabolism to the exact calorie burn, you can visit a doctor's office or training center that is equipped with indirect calimetry equipment, a breathalyzer-like system will give you a more accurate rate. Though I'd never dissuade you from getting the most accurate information as possible, I can tell you that if you have a pencil, a piece of paper, and a calculator (optional), you have pretty much all of the tools to get at least your BMR, which is an excellent start in understanding roughly how much you should be eating.

Now, if you're wondering: Why is ballparking one's *rate good enough*? Don't I deserve better? Don't I want to know it *exactly* my rate so that I don't overindulge and eat too much?

Well, you'd be right. You deserve better. But here's the thing: My diet is more about the quality of foods you're eating and less about the sheer quantity in calories. At the end of the day, calories don't equal nutrients, and I care more about you eating more of the better, fat-melting ingredients contained in this book than I do about seeing you hunched over a desk with a calculator.

Also, if you're engaged in this diet—and sticking to the tasty Super Proteins, Super Fats, and Super Carbs I've laid out—your risk of overeating is severely diminished. You won't be stuffing yourself with bags of greasy potato chips and other cheap eats that will leave you craving even more afterward. You'll find that you're *curbing* your hunger—not increasing it.

After all, you can easily overeat apple-flavored candy all you want and watch your waist balloon in size—but try doing the same thing with *apples* themselves.

Not so easy, right?

That said, knowing your basal metabolic rate is a great start and a solid indicator of generally how much you should be eating on a daily basis. All you have to do is calculate it in just seconds on the back of an envelope using the widely accepted Mifflin-St. Jeor equation.

Here's some easy algebra:

FOR MEN:

10 x your weight (in kilograms) + 6.25 x your height (in centimeters) – 5 x your age (in years + 5).

FOR WOMEN:

The equation is the same, but instead of subtracting 5, subtract 161 at the end.

That's it!

If you're a thirty-year-old woman who stands five foot six and weighs 140 pounds, your BMR is 1,371.75.

But remember: That's your BMR. If all you did was lie on the couch watching *Game of Thrones* all day, you'd be set. So your next order of business is to pile on more calories from there, all of the calories you burn in other aspects of your life.

Let's say you're a runner and you're banging out three miles a day—that's another 300-plus calories (assuming you run nine-minute miles). Very roughly speaking—total ballpark here—you could realistically add another 500 calories for digesting your food, moving around, and cooling down from your run.

If that's the case, you'd be burning upward of 2,200 calories in a typical day. What does that look like? Well, this:

- Three scrambled eggs with peppers and onions
- Cup of Greek yogurt
- Baked salmon and asparagus
- Peanut butter and celery snack
- Chicken, quinoa, and green beans with olive oil

And if the idea of engaging in any algebra whatsoever leaves you in a cold sweat, don't worry! Visit eatthis.com/metabolism-calculator and input your information and we'll do the calculation for you.

SPECIAL REPORT

THE SECRET WEAPON INSIDE YOUR BELLY

Why feeding your microbiome is one of the secret weapons for truly unlocking the body of your dreams.

I HATE TO break it to you, but you're not even human.

Okay, I don't mean that as a put-down, and I don't mean to be a jerk. I actually mean that as fact: Your body is actually home to roughly ten times as many bacteria cells as it is to human cells. Pretty crazy, right? They accumulate on your skin, in your mucus membranes, in your mouth, and all throughout your digestive tract.

Before you get grossed out, know that this isn't just normal—it's super healthy. This enormous but microscopic army of bacterial helpers plays a big role in your life, including your ability to digest food and burn energy. And if you're on a modern-day diet of highly processed foods, it's a good bet you're doing your gut some serious damage.

"In most folks the microbiome is not a healthy place anymore," says Dr. Comite. "It's not healthy because our environment has changed and our gut is the largest organ in our body to interact openly with the environment: the foods we eat, the air we breathe, and the fact that we take antibiotics and our whole structure has changed."

According to her, we're not living off the land like our ancestors did, in which our gut microbiomes would flourish—which is the problem. "We eat so much processed food, we don't really have a healthy microbiome anymore."

The bacteria in your gut have long been thought to serve one primary purpose: aid in the digestion of food, helping you absorb the maximum amount of nutrients and ridding your body of any excess. What's actually going on in your gut is a more delicate dance than most of us recognize, with the specific balance of bacteria in our digestive tract working as the deciding factor in who gets to enjoy an effortlessly fit body and who's stuck trying to shave off the same stubborn weight year after year.

Depending on your genetic makeup, the food you eat, and a host of environmental factors—from the water quality where you live to the pesticides sprayed at your local farm—your gut bacteria can have a beneficial or deleterious effect on your metabolic rate. While we're each born with a unique assortment of gut bacteria, with five hundred distinct species living in our digestive tract at any time, these factors can shift the makeup of what's in our bellies until the bad bacteria start to outnumber the good. The result is a sluggish metabolism and a dramatic increase in the likelihood that you'll become either overweight or obese, even if you're working diligently to eat healthily and get regular exercise. Even worse, once an influx of bad bacteria has invaded your gut, tipping the scales back in your favor can be a difficult proposition without the right tools at hand.

A study published in the scientific journal *Nature* followed obese mice whose high-fat diets were swapped out in favor of more nutritious meal plans. While the mice were able to reduce their weight and lower their blood-sugar levels, pronounced differences remained between the formerly heavy mice and their leaner counterparts—particularly in regard to their gut bacteria.

In fact, the once-obese mice experienced steeper increases in weight when fatty food was reintroduced into their diet, as compared with the mice who had never been heavy. When the slimmer mice had bacteria from the heavier mice introduced into their guts—talk about a procedure!—they experienced the same rapid weight gain as their formerly heavy friends. That's right: The bacteria longed for that formerly heavy time and were eager to send the mice right back to it.

Research conducted at Yale University reveals a similar phenomenon in children: Those struggling with obesity had gut bacteria that worked more expeditiously to turn carbohydrates into fat than their leaner peers. In fact, many of the thinner children studied had no such bacteria to speak of.

In a similar study published in *The American Journal of Clinical Nutrition*, researchers at the University of Turku in Finland found that average-weight children had significantly higher proportions of healthy bifidobacteria, while children who became obese later in life had higher concentrations of *Staphylococcus aureus,* the bacteria that cause staph infections.

While the study subjects' eating habits likely helped shape the proportions of good and bad bacteria in their bellies, genetic factors may play a role in the exact cards we're dealt at birth.

When harmful bacteria take hold in your gut, your weight isn't the only thing likely to suffer. Harmful gut bacteria are linked to the development of leaky gut syndrome, a condition in which toxins borne from your gut bacteria inflame your digestive tract. Once your digestive tract is sufficiently angry, microperforations can develop, allowing those toxic substances to escape their confines and leak out into your bloodstream. This can lead to the development of chronic inflammation throughout your body, and that inflammation, in turn, can slow your metabolism even further.

The good news? Even if your belly bacteria aren't working together in perfect harmony, you're still the captain of this ship; you're the boss of your belly.

The right foods—the unprocessed whole foods contained in

this book—can make all the difference in how fast and effective your metabolism is. Even better, the foods that promote a healthy gut aren't luxury items; they can be picked up at virtually any grocery store. Inulin, a form of prebiotic fiber found in bananas, garlic, onions, asparagus, and Jerusalem artichokes, has been shown to promote the growth of healthy gut bacteria, spurring weight loss and decreasing inflammation in the process.

GET IN SYNC WITH YOUR METABOLIC CONDUCTOR!
HERE ARE THE BEST FOODS FOR YOUR THYROID.

LED ZEPPELIN, Black Sabbath . . . while you may be a heavy metal fan, your thyroid? Not so much. That's because heavy metals, mercury in particular, are chemically similar to iodine—an element the thyroid needs and readily absorbs. When metals like mercury take the place of iodine at binding sites, thyroid hormone production grinds to a halt. The good news is you can instantly detox with fruits that are rich in pectin—a gelatin-like fiber that sticks to toxic compounds in the blood and flushes them out of the body through the urine. In fact, citrus pectin increased mercury excretion in the urine by 150 percent within twenty-four hours of supplementation, according to one study. As a weight-loss bonus, research shows that pectin can limit the amount of fat your cells can absorb. You'll need about four pieces of whole fruit daily to reap the benefits. Whole apples—one of the cornerstone Super Friends in the Super Metabolism Diet—are the absolute best.

Seaweed Your car runs on gasoline, and your thyroid runs on iodine. Insufficient levels of the element inhibit the production of metabolism-regulating thyroid hormones; and since your body doesn't make it, it's an essential part of your diet. That's why, since 1993, the World Health Organization has supported the iodization of table salt. But because recent health headlines have called for the radical reduction of salt intake, some people don't get enough. But you can get your daily dose without OD'ing on salt; there are other dietary sources of iodine, and seaweed is one of the best. Just two tablespoons of brown seaweed or a few rolls of sushi every week will meet your need. And as you nosh on your nori, you'll be blasting fat: Scientists at Newcastle University recently discovered that a compound in seaweed called alginate can suppress the seaweed of fat in the gut.

Brazil Nuts Selenium. No, it's not a Latina popstar. It's the all-essential "on" switch to proper thyroid function—converting T4 hormone into active T3. The essential mineral also protects the gland from inflammatory by-products of thyroid hormone production. Many people who have a sluggish thyroid or thyroid diseases exhibit deficiencies in selenium, and studies show that supplementation can help. Selenium supplementation of 80 micrograms per day—about what you'll find in just one Brazil nut—helped to reduce anti-thyroid antibodies in patients with autoimmune thyroiditis (inflammation of the gland that can make it sluggish if left untreated), one study showed.

Oysters Shuck one for your metabolism. Heck, make it a half dozen. After all, oysters are one of the best dietary sources of zinc—a mineral that's critical, and complementary, to a healthy thyroid. In fact, the body needs enough zinc to activate production of thyroid hormone. And, in turn, we need enough thyroid hormone to absorb zinc. Any way you look at it, deficiencies are likely to result in a sluggish metabolism, and supplementing with the mineral has shown to get weight loss back on track. One study found that obese people who consumed 30 milligrams of zinc per day—the equivalent of just six raw oysters—had improved body mass indices, lost weight, and showed improvements in blood cholesterol levels.

Chicken If your thyroid were a man, he'd be a meat-and-potatoes kinda guy. That's because animal protein is brimming with amino acids, particularly tyrosine—the building block of thyroid hormone, and of dopamine—both of which are necessary for weight management. A lack of tyrosine in the diet may lead to an underactive thyroid, and a deficiency in dopamine is associated with food cravings and weight gain. You can find tyrosine in dairy and leafy greens, but poultry has the added benefit of being naturally low-fat and rich in vitamin B_{12}—deficiencies of which are also common among people with sluggish thyroid symptoms.

Yogurt Every spoonful of yogurt acts as a protective shield for your thyroid. That's because yogurt is naturally rich in vitamin D, and not getting enough of the nutrient puts you at a higher risk of obesity and thyroid diseases, research suggests. Over 90 percent of people with Hashimoto's, an autoimmune disease that's the most common cause of hypothyroidism, are deficient in vitamin D, according to one study published in the *International Journal of Health Sciences. Researchers* say the sunshine vitamin's immunity-boosting and anti-inflammatory properties protect the thyroid from damage. In addition to vitamin D, yogurt is also rich in probiotics that research suggests may help balance "good bacteria" in the gut that can be thrown off by thyroid disturbances.

Chapter 4

HOW THE *SUPER METABOLISM* DIET WORKS FOR YOU!

It's Scientifically Designed to Burn Fat, Not Store It!

BY NOW YOU know that refined carbs, saturated fats, and tons and tons of added sugars and sugary foods are your own personal Kryptonite. These represent many of the popular foods that your body isn't designed to handle and, over time, will lay waste to your metabolism. Also, by now you generally know what foods you should be eating—chiefly Super Proteins, Super Carbs, and Super Fats—if you want to unleash your body's natural superpowers and walk through the world stronger, happier, and leaner.

Are you ready to begin your weight-loss journey?

Excellent. Now, let's get started, shall we?

To recap, the Super Metabolism Diet is divided into two phases. Why two phases? Well, that's simple. At the end of the day, getting your metabolism firing is a simple, two-step process. The first step is to immediately bring to a halt all of the bad behavior you're doing and set your metabolism free. That's part one, the fourteen-day IGNITE phase. During this period, you will adopt a diet that will simply bring your metabolism back up to speed. It's based largely on consuming whole foods while at the same time removing as many processed or prepackaged foods as you can avoid.

When you knock out those baddies, which isn't easy—according to some reports, processed foods account for about half of the modern American diet—you'll not only eliminate any gnarly chemical residue that research shows impacts your endocrine system (which you'll soon learn about) but also you're avoiding all of the useless foods out there that have been stripped of their nutrients (those, too).

Also during the IGNITE, you will eliminate some very specific foods you may reintroduce to your diet later on, including certain grains, beans, nuts, and alcohol. Remember: The IGNITE phase is scientifically designed to activate your metabolism, kick your body's fat-burning mechanism into high gear, and bring your hormones into balance.

Once your metabolism has been IGNITED, you will be amazed to see how quickly you feel a change in mood and your belly fat simply melts away. You'll feel lighter, more energized, happier, and more productive. And you'll still be able to eat all of your favorite foods, plus you'll experience more energy than you've had in years.

And once you've INGITED your metabolism, you will have an understanding of the principles—and have the discipline—to engage in the Super Metabolism Diet for the rest of your life!

Once you've reached fourteen days, you'll switch to the

AFTER BURN phase. In the AFTER BURN phase, you'll continue to incorporate most of the principles from the IGNITE phase, only you'll allow yourself alcohol and other ingredients. And you'll walk through this world knowing that you can always RE-IGNITE your metabolism whenever you want. It only takes about two weeks.

Here are the crucial guidelines for the INGITE phase:

GUIDELINE ONE
EAT THREE FULL MEALS AND ONE SNACK A DAY. (AND REPEAT AFTER ME: "I WILL EAT BREAKFAST EVERY SINGLE DAY!")

IF YOUR BODY is a complex factory that's humming along, you've got to compensate your workers to keep them happily working at peak efficiency. That means ensuring a steady supply of food throughout the day—every day. And if you're eating the right foods—not empty calories or sugary treats—you'll find that it's almost impossible to overeat. That's because when you're eating Super Proteins, Super Fats, and Super Carbs, you'll be feeling full and satiated afterward and won't even want to binge!

And yes, that means eating a breakfast (with protein—more on that later) every morning. I know that a lot of even successful people swear by their practice of eating nothing in the morning. Well, they're not doing their bodies any favors.

In a massive new study published in *The Journal of Nutrition* last September, researchers tracked the eating habits and BMIs of more than fifty thousand adults over the course of seven years and made a compelling case for making a hearty breakfast a cornerstone of your diet. Among other things, they reported something that shouldn't be ignored by anyone who thinks he or she is too busy to start the day with scrambled eggs or a bowl of yogurt and fruit: regular "breakfast eaters" on the whole, the researchers write, "experienced a decreased BMI compared to breakfast skippers."

Ideally, you should have a meal within thirty minutes of waking up. "This will replenish your body from the night's sleep and allow it to function properly throughout the day," says Dr. Matt Tanneberg of Arcadia Health and Wellness Chiropractic. "When you are hungry, your body stops burning calories. That means that your metabolism will dramatically slow down. You need to constantly be replenishing your body's stores to allow it to burn normally."

Here are two samples of what this eating schedule would look like:

SAMPLE SCHEDULE ONE:
A DAY WITH TIER-ONE LEVEL EXERCISE

7 a.m. Breakfast
12 p.m. Lunch
3 p.m. Two-Mile Walk
4 p.m. Super Snack
7 p.m. Dinner

SAMPLE SCHEDULE TWO:
A DAY WITH TIER-TWO OR TIER-THREE LEVEL EXERCISE

7 a.m. Breakfast
9 a.m. 30-Minute Light Lifting Strength Workout or 21-Minute High-Intensity Interval Training (HIIT) Session
10:30 a.m. Super Snack
1:30 p.m. Lunch
6:30 p.m. Dinner

GUIDELINE TWO
STAY HYDRATED—ALL DAY

Superman may have super strength, the ability to fly, and X-ray vision, but according to the comic books, everyone's favorite Kryptonian wouldn't be much good for anything without the sun.

SUPER METABOLISM BOOST!

Small change, big results!

PACK IN SOME PROBIOTICS

What do pickles, sauerkraut, and kimchi have in common? They're all delicious ways to boost your metabolism in a hurry. Researchers at Imperial College London have determined a link between consumption of probiotics, like those found in fermented foods, and metabolic changes linked to decreased fat absorption and weight loss.

That's right: Thanks to the healing powers of sunlight, the man who fights for truth, justice, and the American way is essentially a flying solar panel. You? Well, your powers don't come from above. They come from below.

Specifically: Good old H_2O.

After all, your body is roughly half water. It populates your lungs, your blood, your brain, and your cells. And every single day you lose a lot of it—through sweating, through wastes—and basic dehydration will throw a wrench into countless bodily functions. Consuming enough water is crucial for unleashing the full power of your metabolism. According to a study published in *The Journal of Clinical Endocrinology and Metabolism,* after drinking approximately 17 ounces of water (about two tall glasses), participants' metabolic rates increased by 30 percent. The researchers estimate that increasing water intake by 1.5 liters a day (about six cups) would burn an extra 17,400 calories over the course of the year—a weight loss of approximately five pounds!

Water also delivers crucial nutrients throughout your body, especially to your muscles. Ultimately, it's so important to your body that hydration should be the first thing on your mind when you wake up in the morning. Before you go to sleep the night before, I suggest placing a 16- or 17-ounce glass of water—roughly a pint glass, if you know your beer—next to your bed. When you wake up and go about your morning routine, drink it down.

As your day progresses, you should keep a steady supply of water around you at all times. If you can, invest in a really great water bottle you can keep on your desk or in close reach. The Super Metabolism Diet means you need to consume at least 1.5 liters, or about six cups, a day. If you're engaged in the movement plan, that means more.

One of the best weight-loss tactics anyone can do is to simply cut out any sugary beverages such as sodas—which are also filled with artificial ingredients—and replace them with good old-fashioned H_2O. Now, I know as well as the next guy that's way easier said than done. After all, water can be a bit . . . boring. So here are a couple of quick tips.

First, do what millions of people are already doing: Try drinking more seltzer water (such as La Croix) or investing in a SodaStream device that can add refreshing fizz to your everyday tap water. Carbon dioxide in your water may make you burp, but it contains zero harmful ingredients. (Unless you're literally guzzling it by the gallon, at which point it may cause some damage to the enamel of your teeth.) Second: Keep a big bowl of lemons in your kitchen handy at all times. Not only do they offer a great finishing touch for just about any dish you're cooking, but they're also perfect for adding a healthful twist and injecting a more interesting taste into your *agua* as you make the transition to making the flavorless water a bigger cornerstone of your days.

Whatever you decide to do, here's my general rule of thumb: Start your day with plenty of water, and continually drink to thirst all day long. It should also be the last thing you do before you go to bed.

GUIDELINE THREE
EAT SUPER PROTEINS WITH EVERY MEAL

The Super Metabolism Diet requires you to really pack on the protein.

As I've discussed at length, protein is the fundamental building block of your fat-burning muscle and you need to feed it—

especially if you're incorporating the Super Metabolism Movement Plan. The Super Metabolism Diet requires you to get 1.6 grams of protein per kilogram of body weight every single day. If you're engaged in Tier Three of the Super Metabolism Movement Plan, that number can grow to upward of 2 grams of protein per kilogram of body weight.

Now, what does 1.6 grams of protein (per kilogram of body weight) daily look like?

If you're 120 pounds, that means you weigh roughly 54 kilograms, which translates into about 86 grams of protein daily. You can reach half of that with a half fillet of salmon, which clocks in at roughly 40 grams of protein. Your typical chicken breast has roughly 43 grams of protein. A small steak—let's say 6 ounces of lean beef—comes in at 44 grams of protein. A mere 3 ounces of lean ground turkey yields 21 grams of protein.

But you're not just embracing your more carnivorous side for the sake of your muscles. Eating more protein kicks your metabolism into high gear because your body works hard to digest it—which requires more energy burn. And, because protein is super satiating, you'll find that you won't be overeating as much.

Eating Super Proteins is one of the surest ways to unleash the full force of your metabolism.

GUIDELINE FOUR
CONFINE MOST OF YOUR SUPER CARBS TO THE EVENING

Now, I know this is going to sound crazy to the carbohydrate haters of the world. Yes, the Super Metabolism Diet encourages you to eat good carbs with your meals, but chiefly before bed. Why this heresy?

Well, seventy-eight obese members of the Israeli Police Force recently took part in a six-month randomized clinical trial. The experimental group was prescribed a low-calorie diet (20 percent protein, 30 to 35 percent fat, 45 to 50 percent carbohydrates, 1,300 to 1,500 kcal) that provided carbohydrates mostly at dinner. The control group consumed a similar diet, except that carbohydrate intake was spread throughout the day. After six months, the group eating most of their carbs at night lost slightly more weight and body fat and experienced greater reductions in waist circumference.

Another study in the *European Journal of Nutrition* put two groups of men on identical weight-loss diets. The only difference? Half of the group ate their carbs throughout the day while the second group reserved carbohydrates for nighttime. The result? The nighttime carb group showed a significantly higher diet-induced thermogenesis (meaning they burned more calories digesting their food the next day). Moreover, the daytime-carb group showed increased blood-sugar levels. Another study in the journal *Obesity* saw similar results. Nighttime carb eaters lost 27 percent more body fat—and felt 13.7 percent fuller—than those on the standard diet.

GUIDELINE FIVE
MAKE YOUR FOOD TASTE MORE INTERESTING (AND LOAD UP YOUR SPICE RACK!)

In the sports world, it's called "stacking your team," and it's a tactic that deep-pocketed sports owners know all too well. It's when you overload your team with so many good players that playing the game isn't even fair.

Want to know how the Golden State Warriors knocked off the reigning champs, the Cleveland Cavaliers, in the 2017 NBA Finals, after losing the year before? They shelled out for Kevin Durant, a California newbie who also happens to be one of the best players in the game. Combined with the team they already had on the floor, they were simply unstoppable—finishing the postseason with a mesmerizing 16-1 record.

If you adhere to a diet composed primarily of Super Proteins, Super Fats, and Super Carbs—and make sure you're getting enough water throughout your days starting first thing in the morning—you're well on your way to igniting your metabolism, curbing your cravings, controlling your stress, and getting a much better night's sleep. The dishes in my diet are all packed with those core ingredients. They're the guys already on the floor.

But I've also included a ringer for you to *really* stack the team. Consider this your Kevin Durant.

Science has proven that several meal additions such as peppers, paprika, chili (which all contain the chemical capsaicin), garlic (which supports blood-sugar metabolism, fights inflammation, and lowers blood pressure), and even mustard can help boost your metabolism in small but truly meaningful ways. When you eat these spicy and strong-tasting foods—what any foodie would describe as "better tasting"—you're giving your metabolism an added kick.

A study last year in the *International Journal of Food Science* found that eating chili peppers—whether in a single meal or upward of twelve weeks continuously—does indeed boost your metabolism and "induce weight loss." Its magic ingredient, the aforementioned capsaicin, will up your energy expenditure and spur thermogenesis in your body—also known as the production of heat. According to the study, the chili helps regulate your body's insulin, meaning it literally helps with everything from your blood-sugar levels and weight loss to helping stave off diabetes and heart trouble.

Another study, in the *Journal of Translational Medicine,* discovered that everyday potent ingredients such as cinnamon, cloves, ginger, oregano, rosemary, turmeric, and grains of paradise can actually play a measurable role in helping your body burn fat!

With that in mind, I've stacked the recipes of *The Super*

Metabolism Diet with spices and other taste- and metabolism-boosting ingredients to ensure that your body is operating at maximum burn. Whenever possible, add ingredients such as peppers, paprika, chili, garlic, mustard, cinnamon, cloves, ginger, oregano, rosemary, turmeric, and grains of paradise. Many of the tasty dishes comprised in the Super Metabolism Meals are chock-full of these dietary Super Friends.

GUIDELINE SIX
CUT OUT THE DIETARY SUPERVILLAINS

Immediately eliminate all of these from your diet:

- Breads and cereals (that aren't mentioned in Super Carbs; see page 18)
- Saturated fats (except lean beef and some dairy)
- Alcohol (particularly beer and mixed drinks)
- Refined carbohydrates
- High-fructose corn syrup
- Sodas

GUIDELINE SEVEN
DRINK TEA . . . OR COFFEE!

I know it's hard, but if you always opt for coffee over tea, you could be missing out on a major metabolism boost. In a recent twelve-week study, participants who drank four or five cups of green tea daily, then did a 25-minute workout, lost an average of two more pounds and more belly fat than the non-tea-drinking exercisers. What's its magic? The brew contains catechins, a type of antioxidant that triggers the release of fat from fat cells and helps speed the liver's capacity for turning fat into energy.

But if you stick to coffee only, that's fine, too. Caffeine is shown to offer a small metabolic boost in its own right. Just be sure to drink it black for maximum effect.

GUIDELINE EIGHT
EAT THE SUPER METABOLISM DIET MEALS

In the ensuing chapters you'll find several homemade and easy-to-make meals and Super Snacks that will satisfy your hunger, bring your hormones into balance, and have your metabolism up to speed in no time. Eat them all. Mix them up. If there's one recipe you really love, then, by all means, go crazy and eat it over and over.

If for any reason you're still feeling hungry, don't be afraid to up the portion of Super Proteins, Super Fats, and any of the fruits and vegetables in this book's shopping list!

GUIDELINE NINE
CHEAT!

Once a week during the INGITE phase, allow yourself a cheat meal. Maybe that's a pizza. Maybe that's a burger. Maybe that's a steaming bowl of pasta. Avail yourself of a glass of wine or beer, too, if you like.

But remember: You're working hard to get your metabolism up to speed, so don't overdo it. Because . . .

What One Bad Meal Does to Your Body

WHEN IT COMES to eating for your metabolism, it's helpful to remember that your cells do two things when they receive the stuff from your food: They build things up to store them, usually as fat, and they break things down to create energy. And every facet of my diet is designed so that your factory maximizes the breaking down and releasing while simultaneously minimizing all of that storing. These foods, from the muscle-building, energy-burning Super Proteins to the hunger-fighting Super Fats, will encourage your body to work *for* you, not *against* you.

After all, you're a factory, and I don't want you to have disgruntled employees in your cells storing away fat all day. I

GET YOUR D!

Vitamin D is essential for preserving metabolism-revving muscle tissue. You can nail 90 percent of your recommended daily value (400 IU) in a 3½-ounce serving of salmon. Other good dietary sources: fortified milk and cereal, and eggs. (Also: supplements.)

want you to have a factory that is lean and efficient and churning out energy and burning all of that excess fat.

And for you to do that, it's important to understand what the wrong foods do to your system.

Let's pretend you had a really crummy day at work. Perhaps your boss called an impromptu meeting and you were blindsided by a bunch of questions you weren't prepared for, or you had to give a presentation but you forgot your slides and had to wing it. Whatever the case: You felt humiliated. Hey—it happens to the best of us. (And for more on handling stress, flip to page 135 for my effective collection of Non-Exercise Stress Busters.)

When you go home, what do you do?

I know as well as anyone how easy it is to use a terrible day at the office as the perfect excuse to indulge in some unhealthy foods. You've earned it, right? So let's say you pour a glass of wine and then tuck into a big, greasy slice of sausage pizza.

After you swallow that first bite, enzymes in your digestive system get busy breaking down the carb-heavy crust into simple sugars (or glucose), the proteins in the cheese and sausage into amino acids, and the fats encased in the sausage and olive oil into fatty acids. Throughout your gastrointestinal track, you have the microbiomes—all sorts of organisms that are going to take a lot of these nutrients and, according to Dr. Comite, "they're going to use them in various ways to transport them into the body or to grow or to shrink or to salvage whatever is necessary to make the body healthy." (Your microbiome plays a key role in metabolism, and for more on its importance, turn to page 55.) The broken-down components from your food are then released into the bloodstream, where your hormones come into play.

Now, if your central nervous system works like analog machinery—your brain tells your hand to pick up that slice of pizza through a signal sent directly to your muscles through your body's inner wiring—your endocrine system, the scientific name for your body's hormones, works more like old-school AM/FM radio. Your pancreas, liver, kidneys, and even your fat and your gut, all work like little radio stations creating hormones and releasing them—or broadcasting them—into the bloodstream, where they flow freely through the body until they're picked up again if another part of the body is waiting for them. Your body is, of course, incredibly complex, and there are countless radio stations broadcasting every second, all at the same time. It's how your body's inner factory coordinates and communicates so everyone's on the same page.

As it pertains to your diet, the single most important hormone—the one hormone that essentially hijacks all of the radio waves when you eat—is insulin.

When you eat anything, your insulin, which is produced in the pancreas, immediately rises. As you devour that pizza, your insulin moves into the bloodstream to direct all of that broken-down glucose, amino acids, and fatty acids into your muscles and tissues, where it will be either burned off as energy or stored as fat.

If you eat a healthy, balanced diet, there's no problem eating that pizza. Go for it.

But if you're eating it too often, here's why it's bad for you—and it has almost nothing to do with that tasty sausage or that delicious cheese—after all, most of the amino acids your body can't use simply leave the body as waste—and it has everything to do with the crust.

Excess sugar, refined sugars, and bad carbohydrates are topics I've explored—and, frankly, taken to the woodshed—a great deal over the course of my career, most recently in my last book, *Zero Sugar Diet.*

The truth is that your body has a very complicated relationship with sugar. As it pertains to your metabolism, it's downright dysfunctional. We need sugar to survive, but it's a double-edged sword because the very same thing that we need can also hurt us, balloon our bellies, and send us on the path to diabetes and shorter life spans. For eons, humans relied on sugar—especially your brain, which thrives off glucose—but it was always accompanied by its much more thoughtful companion, fiber. When small amounts of sugar were consumed, usually in the form of whole foods such as fruits, fiber kept that insulin in check.

These days, after the rise of processed foods and refined sugars, we're getting more sugar than we could possibly ever use.

When you flood your bloodstream with too much sugar—especially "free sugars," meaning anything added to the food by a cook, manufacturer, or consumer, plus sugars that are naturally present in honey, syrup, and fruit juices—your pancreas essentially freaks out and releases more and more insulin, and continually hijacks those radio waves.

That army of insulin sucks all of that sugar out of the blood, leading to a condition called hypoglycemia—a sugar crash. Once all of those sugars are out of your bloodstream and dumped into your tissues, your cells can't handle it, so it doesn't get burned off as adenosine triphosphate (ATP)—it gets stored as fat. To make matters worse, the sugar crash triggers an incredible amount of hunger, and the process begins all over again. And when you're flooding your body with too much insulin, too often, you eventually become insulin resistant—when your muscles, fat, and liver cells don't respond as they normally would. This, of course, leads to diabetes.

What drives me crazy about all of these excess sugars is that you're reprogramming your body to be your own worst enemy. Because while you're eating more and more sugars from food, which your body is storing as fat, your body, believe it or not, thinks it's actually starving. Sounds crazy, right? But here's what happens: The fat starts to build up to such high levels that it prevents insulin from working properly in your liver. Your liver's countermeasure is to then release glucagon, insulin's pancreatic alter ego, which, under normal conditions, would ignite lipolysis, the process by which your body takes that stored fat and burns it off. Instead, it turns on gluconeogenesis, the process of making more glucose naturally. So you're making more sugar as well as eating it! Talk about a true double whammy! And when this happens, you're storing so much fat across your figure that your body starts getting really creative.

"By then your body starts to store fat in places it normally shouldn't, like in the liver and in your muscle tissue," says UT Southwestern's Dr. Mangelsdorf. "And when your insulin levels rise higher and higher in your bloodstream, they're problematic for driving cell growth—and not always in a good way. Cancer in particular loves insulin."

Talk about a life-threatening diet.

The truth is that eating a diet high in carbs and sugars will wreck your metabolism. An enormous study published in *The New England Journal of Medicine* looked at 120,877 women and men over a twenty-year period and found that sugar-sweetened beverages, starches, refined grains, and processed foods were the biggest reasons for weight gain—by far. Also, the researchers found that, compared to less processed, high-fiber foods with healthy fats and protein, starches and refined grains are on the whole less satiating. Translation: You're still hungry after eating it, which means you're probably then going to eat a whole lot more.

And if you're eating a diet high in processed foods—frozen dinners, packaged meats, boxed cereals, instant pastas, foods high in margarine, and any other food that has added chemicals, sugars, high-fructose corn syrup, and any artificial ingredients—

you're not doing yourself any favors. Sure, they're wildly convenient, especially if you've got a busy job and more than one mouth to feed every day, but the truth is that, even if they're filled with otherwise "healthy" ingredients—such as fruits and vegetables—there's clear and convincing evidence that they're hurting your waistline and hobbling your metabolism.

In a study published in *Food and Nutrition Research,* researchers from Pomona College in California took eighteen test subjects and fed them either a "whole foods" sandwich, made of whole-grain breads and cheddar cheese, or a processed foods sandwich, based on white bread and processed cheese. In terms of nutrition, the sandwich composition was essentially identical across both types. Though the whole foods one was much higher in dietary fiber, both sandwiches were 15 to 20 percent "protein," 40 to 50 percent "carbohydrate," and 33 to 39 percent "fat." Afterward, they discovered terrible news for the processed foods crowd: Those who munched on the white bread experienced a 50 percent drop in energy expenditure and were a lot hungrier afterward.

Ouch. In metabolic terms, eating processed foods is more thermodynamically efficient compared to eating whole foods— meaning that your body doesn't use nearly as much energy to digest it. Because processed foods contain refined grains, which are ultimately stripped of the bran and the germ and all of the accompanying nutrients—such as B vitamins, phytonutrients, phenols, minerals, and all of that much-needed fiber (basically all of the good stuff), there's not much left for your body to even digest.

At the end of the day, there's little difference between eating that processed snack and eating the box that it arrived in.

So if you're going to unleash the full force of your metabolism, you're going to need to feed your factory with the right substantive foods that will bring it back to life.

THE 20 WORST FOODS FOR YOUR METABOLISM!

Here are the lowliest, sugariest, refined-est, and all-around nastiest foods your body is all but guaranteed to store as fat rather than burn off as energy. Cut them out one by one, and you'll feel better, look better, and walk through life way happier.

---

1) Sugar It probably comes as no surprise that refined sugar is no health food. Sugar causes a serious spike in your blood glucose, slowing your metabolism as your body works to burn it off. Once the sugar has been digested, your insulin levels plummet, making you hungry yet again. Even worse, when sugar isn't burned off, it turns into fat tissue, which burns fewer calories than an equivalent amount of muscle, keeping your metabolism from working as efficiently as it could.

2) White Bread While a single slice of white bread may not be hugely caloric, its ingredients can wreak havoc on your metabolism. The processing used to create white flour robs the wheat of virtually all of its metabolism-revving fiber, and the emulsifiers used to maintain its texture are wrecking your metabolism from the inside out. In fact, research published in *Nature* reveals that emulsifiers had a deleterious effect on the gut microbiome of mice, increasing inflammation along with their risk of metabolic syndrome and obesity.

3) Drink Mixes Think that powdered drink mix is any better for you than a soda? Think again. Drink mixes are little more than a mixture of sugar, flavoring, and artificial colors, the combination of which can cause serious metabolic stalls. Researchers at Talif University found that the consumption of artificial coloring leads to significant decreases in the fuel metabolism of albino rats, making it harder to expeditiously convert food into energy.

4) Bagels Starting your day with a bagel is like putting a stop sign in front of your metabolism. Bagels are little more than a huge portion of white flour with some sugar or high-fructose corn syrup thrown in the mix. Research published in *The Journal of Nutrition* reveals a link between refined grains and an uptick in inflammatory proteins in the bloodstream, making that bagel a serious saboteur when it comes to your metabolism.

5) Soda Most of us wouldn't drink a cup of sugar water, but that's exactly what we're getting when we down a soda. A single 12-ounce can of Coca-Cola packs a whopping 39 grams of metabolism-slowing sugar, 15 grams more than the American Heart Association recommends an adult woman consume in an entire day. With no fiber to temper the sudden blood-sugar surge you'll get from a can of soda, you're looking at a recipe for a slow metabolism.

6) Agave Nectar Agave nectar is often heralded as a healthy alternative to other sweeteners, when, in fact, it's far worse for your metabolism and your health. Agave nectar, while "natural," has a higher fructose content than high-fructose corn syrup—up to 90 percent, as compared to HFCS's average 55 percent—sending your insulin levels soaring and creating the perfect environment for insulin resistance, which can derail your metabolism and make it virtually impossible to lose weight.

7) Nonorganic Produce Organic produce may be more expensive, but that extra cost is well worth it. Nonorganic produce is regularly sprayed with organochlorines, a type of pesticide that has been linked to an increased risk of obesity. The results of a study conducted on newborns in Spain found that those with the highest concentrations of these pesticides were significantly more likely to gain weight rapidly in infancy than those without the chemical in their bloodstream.

8) Artificial Sweeteners Artificial sweeteners may slash the number of calories in your food, but they're also slowing your metabolism. Sugar substitutes can disrupt your gut bacteria, making your metabolism slower along the way. Researchers at the University of Texas Health Science Center at San Antonio found that adult study subjects who consumed artificially sweetened beverages were significantly more likely to gain weight or become obese than those who abstained.

9) Protein Bars That high-protein post-workout snack could be undoing all the hard work you just did in the gym. Protein bars are often loaded with refined sugar, artificial colors, soy, and artificial sweeteners, all of which can contribute to poor gut health and a slower metabolism. All that extra protein is no friend to your health, either; a review of research conducted at the German Institute of Human Nutrition suggests that too much protein can actually have harmful effects on your metabolic rate.

10) Margarine Cutting calories by opting for margarine instead of butter may actually make it more difficult to lose weight. Margarine is often made up of trans fats, which can gum up your metabolism until it's hit a virtual standstill. In fact, researchers at Wake Forest University found that animals given a diet high in trans fats gained more weight than those consuming a diet full of monounsaturated fat, even with no difference in total caloric intake.

11) Blended Coffees The coffee you turned to as a pick-me-up this morning might have just put your metabolism back to sleep. While caffeine is known to have metabolism-boosting effects, when it's combined with huge helpings of sugar, dairy, and artificial flavors and colors, it can still grind your metabolism to a screeching halt. Sugar is known to promote the growth of harmful gut bacteria, slowing your metabolism in the process.

12) Farmed Fish Full of filling protein, fish is generally accepted as a health food, but the differences between wild-caught fish and the farmed stuff are staggering. Farmed fish generally have lower levels of heart-healthy omega-3 fatty acids while packing high quantities of inflammation-promoting omega-6s. Researchers at Indiana University, Bloomington, have also found that farmed fish have higher levels of chlorinated pesticides, which have been linked to lower metabolic rates.

13) Sugary Cereal While cereal is often billed as a wholesome addition to your morning routine, it's often just as bad for you as a doughnut. A single cup of Apple Jacks is not only loaded with metabolism-slowing refined flour, it also packs a staggering 10 grams of harmful gut-bacteria-promoting sugar and some trans fats, thanks to the hydrogenated vegetable oils in its recipe. The result? A metabolic minefield that's sure to leave you hungry again before lunch.

14) Juice If you're giving your kids juice, you might as well give them a glass of sugar and a spoon. While plenty of brands proudly announce that their beverage is 100 percent juice on the label, you're still getting a boatload of sugar in every cup. In addition to all that sugar, which can promote the overgrowth of harmful bacteria in your digestive tract, thus slowing down your metabolism, juice has zero fiber and often packs artificial colors and high-fructose corn syrup, a combination that is a recipe for poor health.

15) French Fries That side of fries you just ordered could be holding you back from the body you want. French fries are often fried in hydrogenated oils, loading them with metabolism-slowing trans fats. Research published in *The American Journal of Clinical Nutrition* has positively linked the consumption of fried foods with an increased risk of abdominal obesity and weight gain in adults, putting your health at risk with every bite.

16) Cocktails Enjoying a cocktail at the end of a long workday does more than just relax you, it relaxes your metabolism to the point that it barely works, too. When you consume alcohol, your body prioritizes flushing it out of your system over digesting your food, slowing your metabolism as much as 73 percent in the process. When you add in the artificial colors and tons of sugar—a whopping 7 grams of the sweet stuff in a single ounce of sour mix—that are mixed in with your booze, you've got a recipe for a slow metabolism.

17) Breakfast Pastries A mixture of white flour, refined sugar, and, in many cases, trans fats, breakfast pastries, like doughnuts, croissants, and Danishes, are no friend to your metabolism. Decimating the healthy bacteria in your gut and promoting an overgrowth of the bad stuff, every time you opt for a breakfast pastry, you're doing a disservice to your metabolism and your weight-loss efforts.

18) Farmed Beef Indulging in a burger from time to time may not seem like a big deal, but if you're eating farmed beef, you could be setting yourself up for a serious metabolic slowdown. Nonorganically farmed cattle are often treated with antibiotics, which can have a profoundly damaging effect on our gut bacteria. Researchers at Harvard found that long-term consumption of diets high in animal proteins can also irreparably alter the balance of bacteria in the gut, slowing your metabolism along the way.

19) Granola Bars Often thought of as a health food, granola and granola bars are one of the sneakiest causes of metabolic meltdowns out there. While their oat base can help lower your blood pressure and cholesterol, the shocking amount of sugar, high-fructose corn syrup, and preservatives in most recipes can make even the most efficient metabolisms slow to a snail's pace. Think your preferred brand is exempt from those unhealthy ingredients? Just a single Quaker Chewy Chocolate Chip Granola Bar is loaded with sugar, corn syrup, brown sugar, corn syrup solids, artificial colors, and the harmful preservative BHT (butylated hydroxytoluene).

20) Frozen Meals What those frozen dinners lack in calories and fat, they more than make up for in metabolism-slowing ingredients. To make up for their lack of flavor, many frozen meals load their recipes with sugar, sodium, and trans fat in the form of hydrogenated oils. The packaging of these foods is just as suspect: many frozen food trays are loaded with BPA (bisphenol A), a chemical used in the production of plastic that has been linked to metabolic disturbances and weight gain.

SPECIAL REPORT

WHAT THE HECK IS HYPOTHYROIDISM?

Here are ten signs that you may have a thyroid disorder—and what to do about it.

CONSTANTLY SLEEPY? Can't lose weight? Does your brain feel like it's in a fog? You may be one of the millions of Americans suffering a chronic, undiagnosed health condition.

It's called hypothyroidism, and it's a condition in which your metabolism-running thyroid gland isn't running at its best. It's sluggish, actually—which is exactly how you feel!

Some thyroid 101 background: Your thyroid gland is the butterfly-shaped gland at the base of your neck that secretes two all-important hormones that control major bodily functions (including how you use energy, regulate body temperature, and digest food) and organs (including the heart, brain, liver, kidneys, and skin). But with hypothyroidism, your body can have normal to low thyroxine hormone levels and elevated thyroid-stimulating hormone (TSH) levels. These high TSH levels are a result of an overworked pituitary gland that is trying to elevate the hormone levels in an inadequately responsive thyroid.

Hypothyroidism is more common than you would believe, and millions of people are currently hypothyroid and don't know it. Because early symptoms of the disease are diverse and mimic the symptoms of everyday life, millions of cases of thyroid disease remain undiagnosed or are mistaken for other disorders. Estimates vary, but approximately ten million Americans have this common medical condition. In fact, as many as 10 percent of women may have some degree of thyroid hormone deficiency, and 12 percent of Americans will develop a thyroid disorder in their lifetimes. With that in mind, here are the signs and symptoms of a sluggish thyroid. Many things can put you at risk for a sluggish thyroid, from genetic predispositions to an autoimmune disorder called Hashimoto's thyroiditis (a condition that occurs in 80 percent of those with hypothyroidism in which the immune system attacks the thyroid). Fortunately, thyroid screening is a simple blood test, and thyroid trouble can often be fixed with the right prescription.

You're Always Tired

Tiredness, constant fatigue, sleepiness, and lack of energy are issues associated with many conditions, but they're strongly linked with hypothyroidism. When it comes down to it, too little thyroid hormone flowing through your blood means your cells aren't getting that "get going" signal, leading you to feel sluggish. Your hypothyroidism may have tricked you into thinking you don't have enough energy for exercise, but actually, by increasing your physical activity, you can help counter fatigue and improve energy levels.

You Keep Forgetting Things

You know you had something to do today, but you just can't remember what it is. Sure, there's sleep deprivation, stress, and aging to blame, but your overall cognitive functioning takes a hit when your thyroid is out of whack. Too little thyroid hormone may cause forgetfulness and poor memory. Because the hormone deficiency slows everything down, neurological functions will also take a toll after some time.

You Have High Cholesterol Levels

Even though your doctor doesn't typically look for thyroid problems during your checkups, he or she will often measure your cholesterol levels. High blood cholesterol levels can put you at risk of getting heart disease, but they also might be indicative of a thyroid problem. According to Reshmi Srinath, MD, "Hypothyroidism causes reduced clearance of cholesterol particles, so LDL and triglycerides may be elevated in a hypothyroid patient."

You've Got No Sex Drive

Having little or no desire to get it on is a side effect of a thyroid disorder. Because of the connection between thyroid function and adrenal glands—the organs that control your "fight or flight" response as well as sexual hormones like testosterone—via the shared hypothalamus and pituitary gland regulators, low levels of thyroid hormone also result in low levels of sex hormones. "Libido is a reflection of testosterone status," explains Dr. Srinath. "Too little thyroid hormone can stimulate a pituitary hormone called prolactin, which then suppresses testosterone levels." While too little thyroid hormone could be a contributor to a low libido, the cumulative impact of other hypothyroidism symptoms, such as weight gain, depression, low energy, and body aches, certainly may also play a part.

You Feel Down

While it might not be a primary symptom, feeling particularly down in the dumps can be a debilitating side effect of hypothyroidism. Dr. Srinath explains that "depression can be related to other symptoms of hypothyroidism such as fatigue, muscle weakness, lethargy, difficulty with focus and concentration." With an underactive thyroid turning many body functions down to low, it's not surprising that your mood might sink, too.

Your Skin Feels Dry

You've bought the face creams, the masks, and the moisturizing lotions, but nothing seems to work. It turns out, dry and itchy skin can be a symptom of hypothyroidism. The change in skin texture and appearance is due to reduced circulation as a result of low thyroid function. A reduction in circulation can cause skin cells to receive one-fourth to one-fifth the normal blood supply, leaving them wrinkled and cracked. Also, a slowed metabolism (caused by too little thyroid hormone production) can reduce sweating. Without the moisture from sweating, skin can quickly become dry and flaky. If just your skin is dry, you could have eczema, but if it is compounded with brittle nails, poor wound healing, and hair loss, you should be checked by your doctor.

You're Struggling to Push It Out

We know constipation is an embarrassing topic that no one likes to discuss, but if you can't boot your bowel issues, it might be time to call up your doctor. Without enough of the metabolism-controlling thyroid hormone, many of your body's functions slow down. One of these functions is the action of the digestive tract, which will start to slow down. Hypothyroidism can weaken the contraction of the muscles that line your digestive tract, causing stool to move too slowly through the intestine. If your sluggish digestive tract isn't due to hypothyroidism, consider eating a banana. The super fruit is rich in fiber to help increase stool weight, potassium to help you avoid bloating and cramping, and prebiotics to help feed good gut bacteria and improve digestion.

Your Muscles Feel Sore—All the Time

We know exercise is a crucial component in reaching your body goals, but it shouldn't be leaving you constantly seeking out a warm bath. If your muscles don't seem to be recovering even on your days off, this might be explained by a thyroid problem. Your thyroid gland secretes hormones that control your metabolism—the body's way of converting the food you eat into fuel. Fewer metabolism-controlling hormones mean a slower metabolism and a disruption in how your body burns energy, which can affect how your muscles feel. To counteract these symptoms, choose low-impact exercises like elliptical-stepping or swimming and increase the consumption of fish in your diet. Fish like salmon are a good source of omega-3 fatty acids, which are known to decrease the inflammation that might be contributing to your muscle and joint pain.

You're Constantly Cold

IF YOU'RE STILL wearing your winter coat when it's 60 degrees Fahrenheit and sunny, you might be suffering from hypothyroidism. It might be easy to adjust the temperature in your house or car, but patients who have hypothyroidism struggle to regulate temperature in their body. Because the thyroid gland controls your body temperature, when hypothyroidism patients' bodies make too little thyroid hormone, body temperature tends to decrease because less energy is being burned by downstream cell targets. Less energy compounded with slow metabolism equals less heat.

Chapter 5

SUPER METABOLISM SUPERFOODS

Eat More, Lose More.

IF THIS BOOK were indeed a big-budget superhero movie and you were the brave hero wearing a cape and cowl, we've officially reached what those in the screenwriting business call a "turning point."

By now, thanks to your sleuth-like powers of deduction and your tireless quest for truth and justice, you've uncovered the true identities of the dietary bad guys—those gnarly supervillains who are hell-bent on bringing nothing short of pain and suffering to your life. You also know that vanquishing them once and for all in a final showdown is the only way to get a happy ending—or a fuller, richer life in which you're leaner, smarter, healthier, more productive, and ultimately happier as a person.

So cue the training montage. It's time to get ready to kick a little bad-guy butt and unleash the full forces of your metabolism!

You know you need Super Proteins, Super Fats, and Super Carbs, but what are they? Well, here you go:

SUPER PROTEINS

Lean Beef: Deficiencies in iron, a mineral, can slow metabolism. Know what's got plenty of it? Lean meat. Eating three or four daily servings of iron-rich foods will help keep your inner furnace burning. Fortified cereals, dried fruit, and dark leafy greens will get you some of the way to meeting your iron goals, but lean meat—with its muscle-building protein content—will be doubly useful in revving up your metabolism.

Also, if you can, opt for grass-fed. Thanks to hormone residues we consume via cage-raised foods, your endocrine system will get thrown out of whack. If you want to give your metabolism a leg up, switch to organic, grass-fed, pasture-raised beef, eggs, and dairy products, thereby avoiding hurting your endocrine system. Also, grass-fed beef is naturally leaner and has fewer calories than conventional meat: A lean 7-ounce conventional strip steak has 386 calories and 16 grams of fat. But a 7-ounce grass-fed strip steak has only 234 calories and 5 grams of fat. Grass-fed meat also contains higher levels of omega-3 fatty acids, according to a

---

SUPER METABOLISM BOOST!

Small change, big results!

GET STRONGER BONES!

Pile on calcium. A study published in *The Journal of Clinical Endocrinology and Metabolism* reveals that women with higher calcium intakes lost significantly more weight—an average of 17.2 pounds—over a four-year study period when compared to those who skimped on calcium.

study published in *Nutrition Journal,* which have been shown to reduce the risk of heart disease.

Eggs: Eggs might just be the easiest, cheapest, and most versatile way to up your protein intake. Beyond easily upping your daily protein count, each 85-calorie egg packs a solid 7 grams of the muscle-builder! Eggs also boost your health: They're loaded with amino acids, antioxidants, and iron. Don't just reach for the whites, though; the yolks boast a fat-fighting nutrient called choline, so opting for whole eggs can actually help you trim down. When you're shopping for eggs, pay attention to the labels. You should be buying organic, when possible. These are certified by the USDA and are free from antibiotics, vaccines, and hormones.

And though it's true that egg whites are low in calories, fat free, and contain most of the protein found in an egg, eating the entire egg is beneficial to your metabolism. The yolk contains fat-soluble vitamins, essential fatty acids, and—most significantly—the B vitamin choline, a powerful compound that attacks the gene mechanism that triggers your body to store fat around your liver. Choline deficiency is linked directly to the genes that cause visceral fat accumulation, particularly in the liver. Yet according to a 2015 National Health and Nutrition Examination Survey, only a small percentage of all Americans eat daily diets that meet the US Institute of Medicine's Adequate Intake of 425 milligrams for women and 550 milligrams for men.

Bison: While grass-fed beef is an excellent choice, bison's profile has been rising in recent years, and for good reason: It has half the fat of and fewer calories than red meat. According to the USDA (United States Department of Agriculture), while a 90%-lean hamburger may average 10 grams of fat, a comparatively sized buffalo burger rings in at 2 grams of fat with 24 grams of protein, making it one of the leanest meats around. But wait, taking a chance on this unexpected meat will earn you two healthy bonuses: In just one serving you'll get a full day's allowance of vitamin B_{12}, which has been shown to boost energy and help shut down the genes responsible for insulin resistance and the formation of fat cells; additionally, since bison are naturally grass-fed, you can confidently down your burger knowing it's free of the hormones and pollutants than can manifest themselves in your belly fat.

Turkey: Lean and protein-rich, turkey is no longer an automatic substitute for red meat–this bird deserves props on its own. A quarter-pound turkey burger patty contains 140 calories, 16 grams of protein, and 8 grams of fat. Additionally, turkey is rich in DHA (docosahexaenoic acid) omega-3 acids—18 milligrams per serving, the highest on this list—which has been shown to boost brain function, improve your mood, and turn off fat genes, preventing fat cells from growing in size. Just make sure you buy white meat only; dark contains too much fat. And know that you're doing your health a double solid by grilling at home: Restaurant versions can be packed with fatty add-ins to increase flavor. Not your problem at home, since it's going straight from the grill to your plate.

Pork: A longtime enemy of doctors and dieters, pork has been coming around as a healthier alternative of late—as long as you choose the right cut. Your best bet is pork tenderloin: A University of Wisconsin study found that a 3-ounce serving of pork tenderloin has slightly less fat than a skinless chicken breast. It has 24 grams of protein per serving and 83 milligrams of waist-whittling choline (in the latter case, about the same as a medium egg). In a study published in the journal *Nutrients*, scientists asked 144 overweight people to eat a diet rich in fresh lean pork. After three months, the group saw a significant reduction in waist size, BMI, and belly fat, with no reduction in muscle mass! They speculate that the amino acid profile of pork protein may contribute to greater fat burning.

Pork and beef run about neck and neck when it comes to protein. But what I love about pork loin is that it cooks so nicely in a slow cooker, barbecued over low heat, or roasted in the oven—methods you should use more often. When you cook meat at high temperatures, and that includes beef, pork, fish, and poultry, chemicals called heterocyclic amines (HCAs) are produced. According to a study in *Nutrition Journal,* increased intake of HCAs causes changes to our gut microbiota—for more on that, see "Special Report: The Secret Weapon Inside Your Belly," on page 55. This increases our risk for colorectal cancer.

Chicken: A 3-ounce cooked chicken breast contains only 142 calories and 3 grams of fat but packs a whopping 26 grams of protein—more than half of the day's recommended allowance.

AND FISH OF ALL KINDS, INCLUDING . . .

Salmon: Salmon may be the best one for your metabolism. That's because most cases of underactive thyroid are due to inflammation of the gland, and salmon boasts significant anti-inflammatory properties thanks to its rich omega-3 fatty acid content. In fact, one study that looked at the effects of weight loss and seafood consumption showed salmon to be the most effective at reducing inflammation—better than cod, fish oil, and a no-fish diet. The fishy fatty acids may also signal thyroid cells in the liver to burn more fat, a recent study published in *The Journal of Nutritional Biochemistry* suggests.

Salmon is among the best sources of fish oil that contains a lot of omega-3 fatty acids. Excellent to raise metabolism and keep your brain and heart healthy.

Tuna: It is a protein bomb that is wonderfully low in calories. And yes, it's good to eat the canned variety. As a primo source of docosahexaenoic acid (DHA), canned chunk light tuna is one of the best and most affordable fish for weight loss, especially from your belly! One study in the *Journal of Lipid Research* showed that omega-3 fatty acid supplementation had the profound ability to turn off abdominal fat genes. And while you'll find two types of fatty acids in cold-water fish and fish oils—DHA and eicosapentaenoic acid (EPA)—researchers say DHA can be 40 to 70 percent more effective than EPA at down regulating fat genes in the abdomen, preventing belly-fat cells from expanding in size. But what about the mercury? Mercury levels in tuna vary by species; generally speaking, the larger and leaner the fish, the higher the mercury level. Bluefin and albacore rank among the most toxic, according to a study in *Biology Letters*. But canned chunk light tuna, harvested from the smallest fish, is considered a "low mercury fish" and can—and should!—be enjoyed two to three times a week (or up to 12 ounces), according to the FDA's most recent guidelines.

Sardines: They're packed with bone-building calcium. Research shows that sardines can improve everything from your cholesterol profile to your mood to your ability to ward off Alzheimer's. Look for sardines packed in olive oil.

SUPER FATS

Avocado: It's like butter that grows on trees. But instead of cholesterol, and trans and saturated fats in butter, avocado contains metabolism-enhancing monounsaturated fat. But that's not all. Each one is also packed with fiber and free-radical-killing antioxidants. Free radicals are destructive rogue oxygen molecules—natural by-products of metabolism—that trigger various chain reactions in the body that destroy cells and DNA, causing all kinds of health problems. Antioxidants in fresh fruits and vegetables can help neutralize some free radicals, but they can't reach the mitochondria—base camp for the free radical army. And that's a problem; when your mitochondria aren't working properly, your metabolism runs less efficiently. Enter: avocado. New research conducted in Mexico found that monounsaturated-rich oil pressed from the fruit can help mitochondria survive attack. Researchers say the results jive with low-disease rates in Mediterranean countries where olive oil—nutritionally similar to the avocado—is a diet staple.

Extra-Virgin Olive Oil: Regularly eating the stuff has been shown to boost levels of adiponectin, a hormone that breaks down fat. Beyond being an ally in the battle against the bulge, EVOO is a go-to pick for total health thanks to its heart-healthy monounsaturated fats. But it's not all good news: Even if you go out of your way to buy extra-virgin olive oil over other varieties, that may not be what's inside the bottle.

Dark Chocolate: Good news for all you chocoholics! Chocolate can help flatten your belly—dark chocolate, that is. Dark chocolate contains the highest percentage of pure cocoa butter, a source of digestion-slowing saturated fat called stearic acid. Because dark chocolate takes more time to process, it staves off hunger and helps you lose weight. Besides the healthy fats, dark chocolate comes packed with antioxidants, principally polyphenols that include flavonoids such as epicatechin, catechin, and, notably, the procyanidins, which can help fight off free radicals and improve blood flow to the brain (which might make you smarter!). A recent study published in the *Journal of Psychopharmacology* found that a few ounces of dark chocolate a day is all you need to reap the benefits.

Nuts: Go nuts! Polyunsaturated fats in nuts activate genes that reduce fat storage and improve insulin metabolism. At about 13 grams per 1-ounce serving, walnuts are one of the best dietary sources (they also have more omega-3 fatty acids than any other nut). A small Pennsylvania State study found that a diet rich in walnuts and walnut oil may help the body respond better to stress and can also help keep diastolic blood pressure levels down. And it's not just walnuts. A study from the *International Journal of Obesity and Related Metabolic Disorders* found that even when two groups of participants consumed the same amount of calories, the group that had more calories from fatty almonds lost the most weight. When it comes down to it, all nuts are great sources of monounsaturated, polyunsaturated, and omega-3 fatty acids, just in varying amounts.

Wild Salmon: Yes, it's a Super Protein and a Super Fat! Salmon might not get as bad of a rap for being high in fat, but its health benefits are worth repeating. By adding this fish fillet into your diet just twice a week, you'll get the full amount of heart-healthy omega-3 fatty acids recommended by the American Heart Association. Omega-3s reduce the risk of arrhythmia, decrease triglyceride levels, and can actually slightly lower blood pressure. When you're at the fish counter, make sure to pick up the right kind—while pink salmon is the second-best fish for nutrition and health benefits, farmed Atlantic salmon is one of the worst.

Flaxseeds and Chia Seeds: Flaxseeds and chia seeds contain a fat called ALA (alpha-linolenic acid), an essential omega-3 fatty acid that can aid weight maintenance and may reduce heart disease risks by promoting blood vessel health and reducing inflammation. A recent review in the journal *Nutrients* found that omega-3s can both enhance fat burning and decrease hunger levels, while a report in *Nutrition in Clinical Practice* found that at a sufficiently high intake, omega-3s improve our ability to metabolize fat by altering the way certain "fat genes" function.

Spirulina: This blue-green alga, available in powders and supplements, is full of healthy omega-3s such as EPA and DHA. Research shows that these forms of omega-3s are more active in the body than ALA at controlling inflammation and belly fat. Not only is spirulina a great source of heart-healthy fats, but it's also super-rich in protein, it's a great source of probiotics, and it may even be able to help flatten your belly during exercise. Nine moderately athletic men took either spirulina capsules or a placebo for four weeks in a study printed in *Medicine and Science in Sports and Exercise*. Afterward, the men who had taken spirulina supplements were able to run 30 percent longer than the men who had taken a placebo, and they burned 11 percent more fat during a run!

SUPER CARBS

Barley: "Barley contains a whopping 6 grams of belly-filling, mostly soluble fiber that has been linked to lowered cholesterol, decreased blood sugars, and increased satiety," says Lisa Moskovitz, RD, CDN. It also has tons of health benefits like decreased inflammation and stabilized blood-sugar levels. And you'll immediately feel lighter. Barley acts as a bulking agent, which can help push waste through the digestive tract.

Whole-Wheat Pasta: You know brown is better, but do you know why? It's because whole wheat contains three parts of the grain, all nutrient rich and fiber-filling. Also try varieties with lentils, chickpeas, black beans, or quinoa.

Sprouted Bread: This nutrient-dense bread is loaded with folate-filled lentils and good-for-you sprouted grains and seeds such as barley and millet. Like quinoa, sprouted bread has been shown to increase the bioavailability of vitamins and minerals. It has this effect on important nutrients like vitamin C, a nutrient that counteracts stress hormones that trigger abdominal fat storage, essential amino acids that aid muscle growth, and belly-filling fiber. Translation: abs for you.

Acorn Squash: Besides serving up a third of the day's fiber, a one-cup serving of this highly nutritious, naturally sweet veggie contains 30 percent of your daily vitamin C needs. The body uses the nutrient to form muscle and blood vessels, and it can even boost the fat-burning effects of exercise, according to Arizona State University researchers.

Legumes: Lentils, chickpeas, peas, and beans—they're all magic bullets for belly-fat loss. In one four-week Spanish study, researchers found that eating a calorie-restricted diet that includes four weekly servings of legumes aids weight loss more effectively than an equivalent diet that doesn't include them. Those who consumed the legume-rich diet also saw improvements in their "bad" LDL cholesterol levels and systolic blood pressure. To reap the benefits at home, work them into your diet throughout the week. Salad is an easy way.

Oatmeal: Yes, oats are loaded with carbs, but the release of those sugars is slowed by fiber, and because oats also have 10 grams of protein per half-cup serving, they deliver steady, ab-muscle-friendly energy. And that fiber is soluble, which lowers the risk of heart disease. The éminence grise of health food, oats garnered the FDA's first seal of approval.

Quinoa: Quinoa is higher in protein than any other grain, and it packs a hefty dose of heart-healthy unsaturated fats. "Quinoa is also a great source of fiber and B vitamins," says Christopher

Mohr, PhD, RD, a professor of nutrition at the University of Louisville. Try quinoa in the morning. It has twice the protein of most cereals, and fewer carbs.

Kamut: Now quinoa, make some space at the table—there's a new ancient grain on the block. Kamut is a grain native to the Middle East. Rich in heart-healthy omega-3 fatty acids, it's also high in protein while low in calories. A half-cup serving has 30 percent more protein than regular wheat (6 grams), with only 140 calories. Eating kamut reduces cholesterol, blood sugar, and cytokines, which cause inflammation throughout the body, a study published in the *European Journal of Clinical Nutrition* found. Toss it into salads or eat it as a side dish on its own.

Chocolate Milk: Why? Well, it's chock-full of protein. Researchers have determined that the ideal protein load for building muscle is 10 to 20 grams, half before and half after your workout. How much protein will you find in low-fat chocolate milk? Eight grams per cup. It also boasts the perfect fat, carb, and protein ratio, as well as the added x-factor courtesy of the chocolate: antioxidants. Add a tall glass of chocolate milk to your morning routine of water and you're looking at a turbocharged metabolism that keeps you burning calories all day long.

Bananas: A bloated belly can make even the most toned stomach look a bit paunchy. Fight back against the gas and water retention with bananas. One study found that women who ate a banana twice daily as a pre-meal snack for sixty days reduced their belly-bloat by 50 percent! Not only does the fruit increase bloat-fighting bacteria in the stomach, it's also a good source of potassium, which can help diminish water retention. Bananas are rich in glucose, a highly digestible sugar, which provides quick energy, and their high potassium content helps prevent muscle cramping during your workout. Each medium banana contains about 36 grams of good carbs: Their low glycemic index means carbs are slowly released into your body, preventing sugar crashes and spurring the process of muscle recovery.

Cherries: Cherries are a delicious, phytonutrient-rich snack. But the true cherry bomb is the tart cherry—not the sort you're used to seeing each summer in bunches at the supermarket. In most of the country you'll find them dried, frozen, or canned. But they're worth seeking out because they are a true superpower fruit. A study at the University of Michigan found that rats fed tart cherries showed a 9 percent belly-fat reduction over rats fed a standard diet. Moreover, researchers noted that the cherries alter the expression of fat genes!

APPLES: Apples are one of the very best sources of fiber, which means you should eat them at every opportunity. A recent study at Wake Forest Baptist Medical Center found that for every 10-gram increase in soluble fiber eaten per day, belly fat was reduced by 3.7 percent over five years. And a study at the University of Western Australia found that the Pink Lady variety had the highest level of antioxidant flavonoids—a fat-burning compound—of any apple.

Sweet Potatoes: The king of slow carbs (meaning they're digested slowly and keep you feeling fuller and energized longer), sweet potatoes are loaded with fiber and nutrients and can help you burn fat. The magic ingredients here are carotenoids, antioxidants that stabilize blood-sugar levels and lower insulin resistance, preventing calories from being converted into fat. And their high vitamin profile (including A, C, and B_6) give you more energy to burn at the gym.

Buckwheat: Like quinoa, buckwheat is gluten-free and a complete source of protein, meaning it supplies all nine essential muscle-building amino acids the body cannot produce on its own, says registered dietitian Isabel Smith. But what makes this relative of the rhubarb such a nutritional rock star is its magnesium and fiber content. "Fiber slows digestion, which wards off blood-sugar spikes and hunger and helps maintain blood-sugar control—all important keys to weight loss and management," explains Smith. Studies have also shown that buckwheat may improve circulation and lower cholesterol.

Potatoes (cold): If you typically eat your potatoes warm out of the oven, you're missing out on the spud's belly-fat-fighting superpowers. When you throw potatoes in the refrigerator and eat them cold, their digestible starches turn into resistant starches through a process called retrogradation. As the name implies, resistant starch, well, *resists* digestion, which promotes fat oxidation and reduces abdominal fat. Since eating cold baked potatoes doesn't sound too appetizing, use the cooled spuds to make a healthy potato salad instead. Instead of buying the drenched-in-mayonnaise deli variety, opt for a vinegar-and-olive-oil-based alternative, which is just as delicious.

Teff: This mild, nutty whole grain is a complete protein that's rich in vitamins and fiber, just like quinoa, says Alexandra Miller, MS, RDN, LDN, a Pennsylvania-based corporate dietitian. What makes it nutritionally superior is its calcium and ab-building iron content. "Teff provides nearly four times as much calcium and two times as much iron as quinoa," says Miller. Don't underestimate these nutrients; their impact on your body is bigger than you would expect. "Diets rich in calcium have been associated with lower body weight and reduced weight gain over time. Calcium also helps keep our bones and teeth strong and may reduce the risk of colon cancer," she explains. Teff can be cooked and added to vegetables, salads, soups, and casseroles, or you can enjoy a bowl of it for breakfast.

Amaranth: Quinoa and amaranth are the ab-carving Wonder Twins of grains. Both are gluten-free sources of complete proteins and have nearly the same amount of fiber and protein. But amaranth has superpowers of its own: "It has more anti-inflammatory monounsaturated fats than quinoa, four times the calcium (an electrolyte that promotes satiety), and 20 percent more magnesium, a nutrient that may aid weight loss thanks to its ability to control blood sugar and ward off hunger," says Isabel Smith. Amaranth makes a perfect substitute for your morning oatmeal. Alternatively, it can be used like quinoa in salads and side dishes.

Greek Yogurt: Packed with protein, crammed with calcium, and popping with probiotics, yogurt has all the makings of the best weight-loss foods. How would you like to take all of the great weight-loss results you've just read about—and double them? That's what happens when you supplement your diet with a combination of vitamin D and calcium, according to a *Nutrition Journal* study. Just four weeks into the twelve-week experiment, subjects who had taken these two nutrients—found in abundance in some yogurts—lost two times more fat than the other group!

Wheat Bran: Packed with bloat-banishing fiber, low in calories, high in muscle-building protein, wheat bran is definitely a nutritional champion. Made from the dense, outer hull of wheat grains, it adds a sweet, nutty flavor to homemade muffins, waffles, pancakes, and breads. It also makes a good addition to hot and cold cereals. If you're really trying to boost your dietary fiber, consume it solo, porridge-style, with a sprinkling of cinnamon and a drizzle of honey.

Triticale: This wheat-rye hybrid will help your six-pack realize its full potential. An able stand-in for rice or quinoa, triticale packs twice as much protein as an egg in a half-cup serving! It's also rich in brain-boosting iron, muscle-mending potassium and magnesium, and heart-healthy fiber. Use triticale in place of rice and mix it with soy sauce, fresh ginger, cloves, shiitake mushrooms, and edamame to make a healthy, Asian-inspired dish. You can also use triticale flour in place of traditional flour in your baking.

BONUS! YOUR SUPER METABOLISM SUPER FRIENDS:

Just like Batman has Robin, you have all sorts of helpers whom you can add to your diet to help you get your metabolism firing. Here are the ones that will give you a much-needed added push.

Tea: Think of your body as a teapot on the stove, and think of the water inside as your belly fat. Chances are the pot is sitting there over a low flame, not doing much of anything. The water inside may be warm, but it's not boiling off. If you want the pot to whistle—and attract a few whistles yourself—you need to crank up the heat.

Well, that's exactly what will happen if you take that teapot from metaphor to reality. Tea—at least, certain types of tea—can rev up your calorie burn as quickly and easily as turning a stove from low to high. Tea can reset your internal thermometer to increase metabolism and weight loss, in some cases by up to 10 percent, without exercising or dieting or sitting in a sauna dreaming about a Nestea plunge.

Just about all tea is good tea, especially green tea, oolong tea, yerba mate, goji, and kola nut.

Spicy Foods: As I mentioned in "Super Metabolism After Dark" (see page 11) and the previous chapter, peppers contain a chemical called capsaicin that gives them those hot-hot-hot properties I love so much! Capsaicin has been shown to speed up metabolism and fight off inflammation. It is found in a variety of peppers that each have a different level of the chemical. Some of the classic favorites are chili, jalapeño, Tabasco, paprika, bell peppers, and habanero peppers (just to name a few). There are plenty of ways to get some of these spicy little peppers into your meals, such as via powders, sauces, or even whole form; but regardless of how you incorporate them, you're sure to get tons of health benefits.

Garlic: Recent studies have shown that garlic supports blood-sugar metabolism and helps control lipid (fat) levels in the blood. Adding garlic to foods that are rich in fats and carbohydrates may keep those substances from doing the damage they're known to do. What's more, eating garlic can help boost your immune system, help ward off heart disease, fight inflammation, and lower blood pressure—to name a few.

Mustard: Add mustard to your meal, and feel the burn—literally! A widely cited study published in the journal *Human Nutrition Clinical Nutrition* found that eating one teaspoon of mustard (about 5 calories) can boost the metabolism by up to 25 percent for several hours after eating. The benefits, researchers say, may be attributed to capsaicin and allyl isothiocyanates, phytochemicals that give the mustard its characteristic flavor.

Apples: A recent study at Wake Forest Baptist Medical Center found that for every 10-gram increase in soluble fiber eaten per day, visceral fat was reduced by 3.7 percent over five years.

Moderate Cheese: You might want to think twice before ditching dairy if you're trying to lose weight, despite what your Paleo-preaching CrossFit friends tell you. Cheese is a satisfying, portable, and inexpensive food that's packed with calcium, vitamin D, and protein. "Calcium can also promote weight loss because it helps maintain muscle mass, which boosts and helps maintain metabolism, helping you burn calories more efficiently throughout the day," says Tanya Zuckerbrot, MS, RD, author of *The Miracle Carb Diet: Make Calories and Fat Disappear—with Fiber!* That doesn't mean you can help yourself to a cheese-drenched casserole, though. Work cheese into fiber-rich snacks to make them more satiating.

Vinegar: Great on salad—and now shown to "switch on" genes that release proteins that break down fat. In a study of 175 overweight Japanese men and women, researchers found that participants who drank one or two tablespoons of apple cider vinegar daily for twelve weeks significantly lowered their body weight, BMI, visceral fat, and waist circumference.

Chapter 6

A GLIMPSE OF YOUR EATING FUTURE

A Seven-Day Super Metabolism Diet Meal Plan

BY NOW, you've learned how to unlock the superpower inside you. In this chapter, I'll teach you how to use it.

Every single day you'll be faced with a barrage of choices you need to make as you navigate on your quest for a stronger metabolism and a healthier body. And thanks to major restaurant chains and the rest of the big-food industry, there are countless traps set along the way to ensure that your efforts get derailed.

Believe me, I know.

I've been studying the science of weight loss for two decades and there are foods out there that only my researchers at Eat This, Not That! can tell you what's inside them. I'm talking about processed foods, foods laced with too much sugar, and foods jam-packed with the worst kinds of fats. I'm talking about easily digestible foods that will elevate your blood sugar and raise your cholesterol and really pack on the pounds.

That's why my goal with *The Super Metabolism Diet* is to make your life as simple as possible. Before every meal, I want you to ask yourself two simple questions:

Am I getting enough protein?
And are my foods . . . Super?

In other words, are your foods on the list of Super Metabolism foods found in this book. Trust me, if you answer those two questions in the affirmative, you will be well on your way to making sure you're eating the right foods to be getting your metabolism firing at full speed. To illustrate how exactly to put the questions into action, let's start at the beginning—with breakfast.

(And if you're eating out, I've also included a list of restaurant dishes from major chains that all qualify as Super Metabolism Diet–approved.)

BREAKFAST. As you know by now, you need to begin your day with a tall glass of water to prime your metabolism for everything to come. Then I would urge you to make one of the dishes in "The Super Metabolism Meals" (see Chapter 9). If you don't have time to make my delicious Jerked Sweet Potato Scramble (page 149), I've included several on-the-go recipes that are easy and come jam-packed with all of the right metabolism-boosting ingredients, including a delicious array of protein-infused Super Metabolism Smoothies and ten super easy oatmeal variations.

If you're still too busy, you can buy a plain Greek yogurt with either added whey or chia seeds for that added protein boost.

And if you must eat at a restaurant, remember, just ask yourself the two questions—am I getting enough protein? And are my foods super? Here are four meals that would qualify:

Potbelly's Egg & Cheddar Cheese Original on Regular Thin Cut

This is the healthiest thing you can get at a restaurant named "potbelly."

410 calories, 21 g fat (11 g saturated), 654 mg sodium, 39 g carbs (1 g fiber, 2 g sugar), 17 g protein

Dunkin' Donut's Wake-Up Wrap with Egg and Ham

America runs on Dunkin', but they'd run faster if they ate more from their new DDSmart menu.

200 calories, 11 g fat (4.5 g saturated), 530 mg sodium, 14 g carbs (1 g fiber, 1 g sugar), 10 g protein—new on their DDSmart menu

McDonald's Egg McMuffin

The Eat This, Not That! Approved classic still packs a protein punch.

300 calories, 12 g fat (6 g saturated), 730 mg sodium, 30 g carbs (2 g fiber, 3 g sugar), 17 g protein

IHOP's Tuscan Scramble

Until IHOP starts offering protein pancakes, this is the best morning meal on the menu.

420 calories, 30 g fat (10 g saturated), 720 mg sodium, 8 g carbs (3 g fiber, 3 g sugar), 30 g protein

LUNCH. If you're prepping some of the meals in this book beforehand—such as the Gangsta Wrap (page 169) (one of my favorites)—you're getting everything you need.

But if you're going to eat a sandwich, don't go for the fatty and sodium-filled deli meats like salami, ham, and roast beef. Instead, swap them out for low-sodium turkey and canned tuna, both of which are extremely rich in protein and will keep you full way past the 3:00 p.m. afternoon slump.

Here're some restaurant examples that could also work, in a pinch:

Panera's Half Cup Low-Fat Chicken Noodle Soup and Half Fuji Apple Salad with Chicken with Reduced Fat Balsamic Vinaigrette

Per serving: 450 calories, 25 g fat (5.5 g saturated), 1,280 mg sodium, 36 g carbs (5 g fiber, 15 g sugar), 24 g protein

Chipotle's Chicken Salad with Black Beans, Fajita Veggies, Fresh Tomato Salsa, and ½ order of Vinaigrette

Per serving: 475 calories, 16.5 g fat (3 g saturated), 1,650 mg sodium, 39 g carbs (10.5 g fiber, 12 g sugar), 42 g protein

Chili's Grilled Chicken Salad

Found under the Lighter Choices menu, this is a grilled chicken breast topped with fresh diced tomatoes, house-made corn & black bean salsa, 3-cheese blend, and honey-lime vinaigrette.

Per serving: 440 calories, 23 g fat (6 g saturated), 1,100 mg sodium, 23 g carbs (4 g fiber, 11 g sugar), 38 g protein

Bonefish Grill's Small Salmon with Mango Salsa, Steamed Asparagus, and Tri-Colored Carrots

Per serving: 440 calories, 31.5 g fat (7.5 g saturated), 930 mg sodium, 3 g carbs, (2 g fiber, <1 g sugar), 37 g protein

DINNER. I know as well as you do how hard it is to eat healthy in the evening after a long, hard day. In 2018, it's never been easier to order up something delicious that will impact your metabolism in all the wrong ways. All it takes is a few keystrokes and the URL "delivery.com."

That's why this is a heroic journey. It requires some level of discipline and sacrifice. But I've taken every conceivable step to make your journey as easy as possible. Not only are the dishes contained in this book super delicious, but they're also easy to make in a short period of time. (No hours-long prep time required!)

If you're making dinner at home "off-menu," remember to ask yourself those two questions: If you're getting enough protein—and you're rounding out your plate with all of the Super Carbs and Super Fats (not to mention the whole vegetables and fruits contained on my complete shopping list)—you'll be setting yourself up for an optimized burn.

However, if you're eating out, whether on a big date or on a business trip, here are some common menu items at major restaurants that fall squarely into my plan:

Chili's 6-ounce Sirloin with Grilled Avocado

Here, you get 100% USDA Choice sirloin with Chili's seasoning and drizzled with spicy citrus-chile sauce, topped with grilled avocado slices, garlic roasted tomatoes, and chopped cilantro. Served with fresco salad. (It's under Lighter Choices in the menu.)

Per serving: 420 calories, 20 g fat (5 g saturated, 0.5 g trans), 1,610 mg sodium, 23 g carbs (6 g fiber, 7 g sugar), 39 g protein

Applebee's Pepper-Crusted Sirloin and Whole Grains

From the lighter fare menu: pepper-crusted sirloin on a bed of hearty whole grains with sautéed spinach, fire-roasted grape tomatoes, and portobellos, finished with a light broth.

Per serving: 380 calories, 13 g fat (4 g saturated), 1,850 mg sodium, 38 g carbs (6 g fiber, 7 g sugar), 30 g protein

PF Chang's Buddha's Feast Steamed and a half order of Small Brown Rice

Five-spice tofu, savory sauce, asparagus, shiitakes, broccoli, carrots.

Per serving: 440 calories, 4 g fat (0 g saturated), 300 mg sodium, 72 g carbs (12 g fiber, 11 g sugar), 30 g protein

Red Lobster's Lighthouse Rock Lobster Tail with Rice and Broccoli

Wild-Caught Caribbean Lobster, wood-grilled, and served with rice and fresh broccoli.

Per serving: 450 calories, 15 g fat (3 g saturated), 1,260 mg sodium, 35 g carbs (4 g fiber, 4 g sugar), 45 g protein

Outback Steakhouse's Victoria's 6-ounce Filet Mignon with Steamed Broccoli and Side House Salad with Light Balsamic

Per serving: 505 calories, 30 g fat (11 g saturated), 1,350 mg sodium, 34 g carbs (8 g fiber, 16 g sugar), 51 g protein

Olive Garden's Herb-Grilled Salmon with Garlic-Herb Butter and Parmesan-Garlic Broccoli

Filet "grilled to perfection" and topped with garlic-herb butter. Served with parmesan-garlic broccoli.

Per serving: 460 calories, 28 g fat (8 g saturated), 570 mg sodium, 8 g carbs (4 g fiber, 3 g sugar), 43 g protein

TGI Friday's Mediterranean Shrimp Naan

They call this one "Grilled shrimp drizzled with balsamic glaze and served on naan bread with cucumber yogurt sauce, mixed greens, and garlic, basil, and tomato bruschetta."

Per serving: 470 calories, 15 g fat (3.5 g saturated), 1,260 mg sodium, 54 g carbs (4 g fiber, 6 g sugar), 31 g protein

Now, that said, here's an example of how you can structure a full week of eating. It's not written in stone, by any means: Mix up the meals. Substitute meals wherever you feel like it—or simply eat the same thing over and over. Whatever you want! The purpose of this chart is simply to show you how to follow the principles of *The Super Metabolism Diet*.

MONDAY

When you wake up: Tall glass of water (16 ounces)

Breakfast: Quiche "Muffin" (see page 146)

Snack: One red apple

Lunch: Grilled chicken breast in a whole-wheat pita, with lettuce, tomato, avocado, and Dijon mustard

Dinner: Indian Stir-fry with Blistered Green Beans (see page 185)

TUESDAY

When you wake up: Tall glass of water (16 ounces)

Breakfast: Bowl of oatmeal with chia seeds and banana

Lunch: Steak salad, with radishes, carrots, arugula, tomatoes, and olive oil

Snack: Three slices of deli turkey; one peach

Dinner: Hazelnut-crusted Salmon (with Wilted Kale) (see page 180)

WEDNESDAY

When you wake up: Tall glass of water (16 ounces)

Breakfast: Two eggs fried in olive oil; side of turkey bacon

Snack: Greek yogurt with fruit

Lunch: Pho-style Turkey Lettuce Wraps (see page 164)

Dinner: Grilled Skirt Steak with Olive Tzatziki (see page 182)

THURSDAY

When you wake up: Tall glass of water (16 ounces)

Breakfast: Buenos Días Black Beans (see page 150)

Snack: Carrots and hummus

Lunch: Niçoise farro salad

Dinner: Weeknight Penne with Veggies and Chicken Sausage (see page 184)

FRIDAY

When you wake up: Tall glass of water (16 ounces)

Breakfast: Loaded Breakfast Sausages (see page 153)

Lunch: Vintage Tuna-Tomato Salad (see page 162)

Snack: One red apple

Dinner: Grilled Caesar Salads with Avocado Dressing (see page 175)

SATURDAY

When you wake up: Tall glass of water (16 ounces)

Breakfast: Greek yogurt with a side of berries

Snack: Hot-Chilly Super Smoothie (see page 163)

Lunch: Turkey

Dinner: Sheet-Pan Pork (with Roasted Cauliflower and Onions) (see page 178)

SUNDAY

When you wake up: Tall glass of water (16 ounces)

Breakfast: Jerked Sweet Potato Scramble (see page 149)

Lunch: Arugula with Asparagus Bundles and Whirled Mango (see page 165)

Snack: One serving of bison jerky

Dinner: Riced Cauliflower and Shrimp Tabbouleh (see page 174)

BE A SPICE GIRL . . . OR GUY!

Some great spice blends you can add to any meal to help you boost your metabolism.

CINNAMON AND SUGAR:

◼ While cinnamon and sugar team up as well as peanut butter and jelly, the sweet spice combo serves up way more benefits than your favorite childhood sammy. Sugar almost always elevates blood-sugar levels (uh, duh!), but cinnamon boasts the heaven-sent powers of its polyphenols, which help stabilize blood sugar and shoo away pesky insulin spikes. Wanna hear something even sweeter? An animal study published in the *Archives of Biochemistry and Biophysics* reported that adding cinnamon to participants' diets resulted in decreased belly fat.

GINGER AND MATCHA:

◼ Ginger, just like matcha green tea, has been shown to de-bloat the tummy. And matcha especially has been praised for blessing its drinkers with bikini-ready bodies. In fact, a Taiwanese study revealed that participants who regularly drank the green tea had nearly 20 percent less body fat than the non-imbibers. And in a Swedish study, people who replaced water with green tea noticed reduced hunger compared to those who didn't fill up on the stuff. So what's the secret? EGCG (epigallocatechin gallate), a metabolism-boosting nutrient in green tea, amps up the breakdown of fat while blocking fat-cell formation.

COCOA AND CHILI:

◼ Believe it or not, the main ingredient in your favorite bar of dark chocolate packs in some serious punch. Plenty of studies show that cocoa can help control diabetes, liver cirrhosis, and even Alzheimer's. Plus, a study printed in the journal *Circulation: Heart Failure* revealed that women who enjoyed just one to two servings of high-quality chocolate on a weekly basis had a 32 percent lower risk of developing heart failure than their non-indulging counterparts. By adding some chili to it, not only will it amp up your chocolate's flavor, but it'll also lend it some serious flat-belly benefits. After all, it's got capsaicin.

CAYENNE AND CUMIN:

■ Fiery cayenne is actually pure chili that's ground up from the emoji-inspiring cayenne chili pepper. So, it may not surprise you that it's a great weight-loss effort-booster. Just as mentioned above, capsaicin (found in cayenne) has been proven to reduce abdominal fat by controlling appetite and boosting the body's thermogenesis (its ability to burn food as energy).

And . . .

JUST JALAPEÑOS:

■ The jalapeño pepper is one of the top heat-lover favorites! When eaten, it gives a warm burning sensation that aids weight loss and has disease-fighting properties.

Chapter 7

GET THE BEST NIGHT'S SLEEP— EVER

Optimize Your Body's Inner Reboot, and Prime Your Metabolism to Fire Every Day

IF YOU STEPPED in a time machine and asked a twenty-two-year-old version of me, when I first embarked on a life-long career in the world of healthy living and self-improvement, what the biggest dangers to your health are, I could've easily reeled off the usual suspects. You know— smoking, lack of exercise, eating the wrong foods. Years later, of course, those baddies are still as bad as ever. But I couldn't have predicted when I started out in the early 1990s that one of the most insidious forces on your health in 2018 would be something so pervasive that it's downright inescapable: light.

No, not the beautiful kind that rains down vitamin D from the sky. I'm referring to a very specific type of artificial light, or "blue" light, the kind that is emitted by everything from your new eco-friendly lightbulbs to the display interface on your iPad. At first, I was truly skeptical about the harmful effects of artificial light in our lives. After all, like most Americans, I grew up with a television set forever in close reach. To this day, I'm known to watch an episode or two of *Family Guy* before calling it a night. And, truth be told, human beings have always had ways of extending their days into the wee hours, whether they're burning wood, gas, or whale blubber. In a world where obesity is rampant and heart disease remains one of the biggest killers of them all, don't we have bigger fish to fry than the lighting in your bedroom?

Well, more and more we're learning that our artificially illuminated world is simply devastating our sleep. When you check your email in bed before going to sleep—or you dive into that new Grisham novel on your iPad—and the shorter-wavelength (or "blue") light hits the photosensitive cells in your eye, it effectively slows the release of "sleep-promoting" neurons and "activates arousal-promoting" neurons. It suppresses the release of melatonin, the brain's chemical for making you sleepy.

Oh, and speaking of that melatonin? After you turn thirty years old, your levels start to fall, making going to bed that much tougher.

If you talk to leading researchers and sleep activists like Charles Czeisler FRCP, PhD, MD, and head of the Harvard Medical School Division of Sleep Medicine—who works with several professional sports teams on their sleep schedules—we're in the middle of nothing short of a modern sleep crisis. According to Czeisler, the ubiquity of smartphones, tablets, and even eco-friendly lightbulbs is keeping humans up later and later, and we're all shifting our time zones forward into the wee hours while still forcing ourselves out of bed early in the morning. The result? Not just less sleep, but also *terrible* sleep. And when you're getting less and terrible sleep, you're obviously tired, you're less active, and the vicious cycle of weight gain begins. Our current awareness of the importance of sleep, says Czeisler, is on par with our awareness of smoking in the 1950s.

"The light sources are getting brighter and worse," he told us in a report I commissioned for *Men's Fitness*.

Aside from the obvious dangers—according to its "conservative" estimate, the National Highway Traffic Safety Administration estimates at least 100,000 "police-reported" crashes due to driver fatigue every year, resulting in 1,550 deaths, 71,000 injuries, and $12.5 billion in losses—there are massive health concerns, as well. According to the Centers for Disease Control and Prevention, getting less *z*'s is associated with diabetes, heart disease, depression, and obesity. In 2014, researchers published the findings of a five-year study of the sleep cycles of 13,742 participants in the journal *Obesity*, which found that there is a direct correlation between sleep duration and waist circumference (and body mass). "Compared to participants who reported sleeping 7–9 hours a night," the researchers concluded, "short sleepers [or those who log less than six hours of sleep per night] were more likely to be obese and have abdominal obesity."

A lot of my friends—especially the ultracompetitive types who work long hours in the financial sector—love nothing more than to brag about how little they need to sleep. Well, the truth is that they're wrong. According to the National Sleep Foundation, only 4 percent of adults actually qualify as "short sleepers"—or those who can function on fewer than five hours per night. And more and more we're learning that sleep isn't just "rest," and it's more important than we ever imagined.

A few years ago, researchers published a landmark study in the journal *Science* that advanced our knowledge of sleep by nearly a generation. We've always known that sleep is important, but we've never really known why. Well, the study revealed that one of the primary reasons we sleep is simple waste removal. You may recall that I said you have trillions upon trillions of cells in your body. But as you grow older, your body is constantly replacing them all the time. Cells die, they multiply. It's normal. Like fat cells, our brain cells, according to Czeisler, are different, because the connections are so complicated and "because our memories are stored in those connections." Sleep, the researchers discovered, is your body's process for shutting down so that you actually can clean those cells of toxins using your spinal fluid. It's an actual *physiological* process. "When you sleep, the space between the [brain] cells becomes larger," says Czeisler. "There is a structural change, with things moving in relation to one another. It would be as if all the buildings in Manhattan shrank, and the alleys and streets got bigger for the garbage trucks. It was remarkable."

Think about that: If you're not sleeping, you're walking around with a toxin-infested brain. And every day that you're walking the world under-slept, you'll actually be experiencing very mild forms of hallucination. In a recent German study of under-slept night-shift nurses, researchers found that the participants repeatedly failed visual perception tests. When rested, of course, they passed with flying colors.

Also, it's important to remember that as you sleep, you may be unconscious and your metabolism slows, but your factory is still very, very much alive. Your sleep is your reboot period, when your body rebuilds and repairs its cells throughout your body—as well as your all-important muscles. It's when your cortisol starts to build so you can be alert in the morning and when your body fortifies its immune system.

Research has shown that lack of sleep throws off your hormonal balance. A study by the University of Wisconsin medical school found that those who routinely slept only five hours a night awoke to find that their ghrelin levels (the hormone that tells you to eat) were nearly 15 percent higher—and their leptin levels (the hormone that tells you when you're full) were nearly 16 percent lower—than people who slept a full eight hours. If you need me to spell that out for you, here you go: Not getting enough sleep means you're literally reprogramming your body to switch off the satiating function and turn on the floodgates for the hunger function.

Talk about a one-way ticket to belly fat.

And have you ever woken up with a killer hangover? Well, you're dehydrated, and likely have a terrible headache alongside nausea and even diarrhea. But there's also another ghastly side effect to knocking back a few too many glasses of wine or tequila at the bar: You've destroyed your sleep.

At first, this may seem counterintuitive. If you've had plenty to drink, you know as well as anyone how easy it is to *fall* asleep. But that's about the only good news from the connection between booze and z's. First of all, alcohol throws off your natural sleep rhythms. According to the National Sleep Foundation, a booze-filled brain means you're turning on "alpha activity," which is a brain state that doesn't normally occur during sleep but rather when you're "resting quietly." Combine that with the slow-wave deep sleep—also known as delta activity, which is crucial for consolidating memories—and you're busting up your mind's attempt to restore itself.

You're also guaranteed to wake up too early.

Ever had a few cocktails and then hit the sack, only to bolt out of your slumber way earlier than you wanted to?

When you've been drinking, your body quickly produces adenosine, a chemical that lulls you to sleep quickly. But it goes away just as quickly, meaning you're all but guaranteed to pop out of bed without sufficient rest. Throw in the fact that alcohol disrupts your all-important REM (rapid eye movement) sleep—when your brain sets about restoring itself—causes sleep apnea, and largely makes you pee a ton, and you're looking at a recipe for a tired, groggy, and hungry day.

That's why the diet plan contained in this book takes a hard look at your alcohol intake.

HOW TO GET A BETTER NIGHT'S SLEEP—GUARANTEED!

Drop pounds and lose belly fat with the help of these simple p.m. hacks.

What's the best place in the world to lose weight? *The gym!* say the muscle-bound personal trainers. *The track!,* say the distance runners, cyclists, triathletes, and other types trucking along with sweat in their eyes and numbers stuck on their chests. *The kitchen!* say the nutritionists, dieticians, and organic-produce purveyors.

Though they're not entirely wrong, if you want real, successful, and sustainable weight loss, it actually comes from another place, as well: *the bedroom!*

No, you can't lovemake your way to being lean. But you can absolutely sleep your way to a slimmer you. In fact, no matter how many pounds you press, how many miles you log, how much kale you crunch, it won't get you anywhere near your weight-loss goals unless you're also getting enough quality sleep. Here are a few simple tweaks to your p.m. routine that can mean serious weight-loss success.

GIVE SNOOZE ITS DUE

■ To turn sleep into prime weight-loss time, realize how important a good night's sleep is for optimizing and regulating all of your bodily functions, including how you use and store caloric energy. The hormones at play here are leptin and ghrelin. Leptin helps to regulate your energy levels and keep your appetite low, while ghrelin stimulates hunger and often initiates the need to eat. People who get more sleep have reduced ghrelin and increased leptin levels, which helps to control their appetites throughout the day. That was the finding of research conducted at the University of Wisconsin. Another study published in the *Archives of Internal Medicine* found that overweight people, on average, got sixteen minutes less sleep per day than people of regular weight. Although that might not sound like a big difference, those minutes—like your belly fat—accumulate over time.

HAVE A CUP OF TEA

■ Wind down with a cup of rooibos tea, and burn belly fat while you do it! Naturally decaffeinated, rooibos tea is made from the leaves of the "red bush" plant, grown exclusively in South Africa. What makes rooibos tea particularly good for your belly is a unique and powerful flavonoid called aspalathin. Research shows that this compound can reduce stress hormones that trigger hunger and fat storage.

TRIP YOUR SLEEP SWITCH

■ Don't count sheep, eat lamb! (Or better yet, a bit of turkey.) Tryptophan, an amino acid found in most meats, has demonstrated powerful sleep-inducing effects. A recent study among insomniacs found that just ¼ gram—about what you'll find in a skinless chicken drumstick or 3 ounces of lean turkey meat—was enough to significantly increase hours of deep sleep. And that can translate into an easy slim-down. Researchers from the University of Colorado found that dieters consumed 6 percent fewer calories when they got enough sleep. For someone on a 2,000-calorie diet, that's 120 calories per day, which could amount to nearly a one-pound weight loss in a month! The National Sleep Foundation suggests seven to eight hours of sleep for most adults.

EAT COTTAGE CHEESE

■ Completely avoiding food before bedtime can actually be bad for your weight-loss goals. First, going to bed with a rumbling tummy makes falling asleep difficult. Second, people who wake up feeling hungry are far more likely to pig out on a big breakfast. Have a little cottage cheese before bed. Not only is it rich in casein protein, but it also contains the amino acid tryptophan.

CREATE A ROUTINE

■ By doing the same thing every night, for at least an hour before bedtime, you're actually programming sleep triggers. These triggers could include writing in your sleep diary or having a cottage cheese snack, or indeed any other items from this list. Over time, your brain will begin to associate those things with bedtime and fast-track you into fat-burning slumber.

OBSERVE STRICT KITCHEN HOURS

■ Nighttime fasting—a.k.a. closing the kitchen early—may help you lose more weight, even if you eat more food throughout the day, according to a study in the journal *Cell Metabolism*. Researchers put groups of mice on a high-fat, high-calorie diet for one hundred days. Half of them were allowed to nibble throughout the night and day on a healthy, controlled diet, while the others had access to food for only eight hours but could eat whatever they wanted. The result of the sixteen-hour food ban? The fasting mice stayed lean, while the mice who noshed 'round the clock became obese— even though both groups consumed the same amount of calories!

DO A LITTLE WEIGHT LIFTING

■ Pre-sleep resistance training can really help to optimize the weight you lose during sleep. According to an article published in the *International Journal of Sport Nutrition and Exercise Metabolism*, subjects who performed resistance exercises enjoyed a higher resting metabolic rate for an average of sixteen hours following their workout. If you usually work out first thing in the morning, your sleepy-time weight loss won't be impacted by that spike in metabolism. Go big, go home, then get into bed.

RELAX

■ There's nothing more frustrating than looking at the clock all night and cursing yourself for not being able to drift off at 1:00 a.m., 2:00 a.m., and again, at 3:00 a.m. It certainly doesn't help things. Take comfort in the fact that merely relaxing your mind and body will help rejuvenate you in lieu of honest-to-goodness sleep. Once you're not so excited about your inability to fall asleep, it'll come more naturally.

FOLLOW THE TWENTY-MINUTE RULE

■ If you're not getting anywhere after chilling out for twenty minutes, get out of bed, leave the bedroom, and do something quiet and unstimulating. Try reading a book or flipping through a catalog.

SHAKE THINGS UP

■ Having a protein shake before hitting the sack may boost your metabolism, according to one Florida State University study. Researchers found that men who consumed good snacks in the evening that included 30 grams of either whey or casein protein had a higher resting metabolic rate the next morning than when eating nothing. Protein is more thermogenic than carbs or fat, meaning your body burns more calories digesting it.

DO SOME SIMPLE BODY-WEIGHT EXERCISES OR SOME LATE CARDIO

■ Maybe the rigmarole of getting dressed and going to the gym after dark isn't for you, and that's understandable. But that doesn't mean you can't use your body weight for a quick workout before bed. According to *Combat the Fat* author Jeff Anderson, body-weight exercises target muscles in a unique way due to the effect of fighting gravity. Examples of these exercises include push-ups, pull-ups, dips, and body-weight squats.

Examples of cardio include walking around the neighborhood, walking or running up and down the stairs, and jogging and/or riding an exercise bike. Adding activities like these to your pre-bed routine can help you to burn belly fat. Bonus points if you can do a little resistance training immediately before your late cardio session. Studies show that cardio is more effective if you do it immediately after weight lifting or body-weight exercises.

MAKE A TO-DO LIST

■ Thoughts of a busy day whizzing around your head won't help you get in the right condition for a relaxing eight-hour sleep shift. Try writing down everything you need to do the next day. It can make your life seem more manageable.

LET THE COLD AIR IN

■ A striking new study published in the journal *Diabetes* suggests that simply blasting the air conditioner or turning down the heat in winter may help us attack belly fat while we sleep. Colder temperatures subtly enhance the effectiveness of our stores of brown fat—fat keeps you warm by helping you burn through the fat stored in your belly. Participants spent a few weeks sleeping in bedrooms with varying temperatures: a neutral 75 degrees, a cool 66 degrees, and a balmy 81 degrees. After four weeks of sleeping at 66 degrees, the subjects had almost doubled their volumes of brown fat. (And yes, that means they lost belly fat.)

TAKE A BATH OR A SHOWER

■ A UCLA study of some of the world's last remaining hunter-gatherer tribes noted that temperature drops were an important sleep cue for our Paleolithic forebears. We no longer sleep under the stars that much, but you can re-create a sunset-like temperature drop by taking a hot bath or shower. The dip might make your pound-shedding shut-eye deeper and make you fall asleep faster.

MAKE A MINT

■ Certain scents can make your mouth water, and others can actually suppress your appetite. One study published in *The Journal of Neurological and Orthopaedic Medicine* found that people who sniffed peppermint every two hours lost an average of five pounds a month! Banana, green apple, and vanilla had similar effects. Consider burning a minty candle until you head to bed to fill the room with slimming smells. If you don't want to bother with blowing out candles before you turn down the covers, try adding a few drops of peppermint oil to your pillow.

TURN OUT THE LIGHTS EARLY (INCLUDING YOUR DEVICES)

■ Exposure to light at night doesn't just interrupt your chances of a great night's sleep, it may also result in weight gain, according to a new study published in the *American Journal of Epidemiology.* Study subjects who slept in the darkest rooms were 21 percent less likely to be obese than those sleeping in the lightest rooms.

As previously discussed, the more electronics we bring into the bedroom, the fatter we get—especially among children. A study in the journal *Pediatric Obesity* found that kids who bask in the nighttime glow of a TV or computer don't get enough rest and suffer from poor lifestyle habits. Researchers found that students with access to one electronic device were 1.47 times as likely to be overweight as kids with no devices in the bedroom. That increased to 2.57 times for kids with three devices. Even if you're a full-grown adult, it's best to leave your iPad in the living room.

If you're addicted to your smartphone—use an app like f.lux to reduce the blue light emitting from your computer and smartphone. It works by eliminating eye strain from the harsh light that inhibits melatonin production. Melatonin is the hormone responsible for regulating sleep rhythms. Some newer iPhones and iPads have a similar built-in feature called Night Shift.

EAT SOME CARBS—SERIOUSLY

■ Eating carbs before bed may not be a bad idea if you want to lose some weight! Seventy-eight obese members of the Israeli Police Force took part in a six-month randomized clinical trial. The experimental group was prescribed a low-calorie diet (20 percent protein, 30–35 percent fat, 45–50 percent carbohydrates, 1,300–1,500 kcal) that provided carbohydrates mostly at dinner. The control group consumed a similar diet, except that carbohydrate intake was spread throughout the day. After six months, the group eating most of their carbs at night lost slightly more weight and body fat and experienced greater reductions in waist circumference.

STRIKE A POSE

■ By the time you've had your time on this mortal coil, you'll have spent up to thirty years asleep. To get the most out of that investment, you'd better figure out which sleeping posture you find most restorative, then build your bed around it. You can do that by buying the right mattress and pillow to mitigate against any areas of discomfort. If you sleep on your side, putting a pillow between your legs will minimize twisting strain on your lower back, while hip pain can be lessened by using a mattress topper to help soften and contour your body.

START A SLEEP DIARY

■ Do you really have an accurate read on how much sleep you are or aren't getting? It's always best to work from data, even if you're the one logging the quality and duration of your sleep. Simply list each complete hour you were asleep in bed, and each partial hour (including naps). Then make a note of the events that may have influenced your sleep. Did you exercise that day? Drink a lot of coffee? After two weeks, read through the whole thing, looking for patterns. The results may surprise you—and help you with your weight-loss goals.

EAT PEPPER

■ Scientific studies have shown that one of the most effective ways to burn fat is to eat peppers. Your body continues to burn fat while you sleep as a direct result of including them with your meals. If it works with your palate, include a little with your cottage cheese snack.

BREATHE THROUGH YOUR NOSE

■ Why? Well, first it will prevent snoring. That will not only improve your sleep but also the sleep of anybody else in earshot. Secondly, it provides more oxygenation, so you can take those deep breaths that help to relax the body. Use Breathe Right strips if you're stuffy.

LEARN YOUR CIRCADIAN RHYTHM

■ Pay attention to the times you feel and perform at your best, when you naturally wake without an alarm clock, and when you start to feel sleepy in the evenings. Add this info to your sleep diary. This information will tell you about your "chronotype," which will allow you to set healthy sleep goals that work with your natural rhythms. A free online assessment at the Center for Environmental Therapeutics can help you find your type and provide related advice.

KEEP EATING!

■ Nutrient-dense meals frequently throughout the day serve to keep your metabolism ticking and will ensure that your body continues burning fat throughout the night. Furthermore, eating frequently will ensure that your appetite is kept in check, which will reduce any cravings you have when you wake.

Chapter 8

TAKE CONTROL OF YOUR STRESS

It's One of the Deadliest Metabolism Killers of Them All. Not Anymore. Reboot, and Prime Your Metabolism to Fire Every Day.

LET ME GUESS. When you hear the word "stress," the first thing that pops into your mind is an image of you hunched over your desk at work—sweating profusely—with a clock loudly ticking in the background, a deadline looming, and your body temperature rising so fast you start to sweat. Or maybe you imagine yourself stuck in traffic, fifteen minutes late for an important job interview—or late to pick up your kids from school—and you start pounding the steering wheel and cursing. Trust me, we've all been there, and that stress is terrible for your health. And god knows that we are, as a people, undeniably feeling the harsh pressures of work.

According to data compiled by the Department of Safety, Security, and Emergency Management at Eastern Kentucky University, being a working professional in America means living your life at peak misery—and it's only getting worse.

It cited loads of cutting-edge research, including a study that polled twenty-six thousand Americans across the country and found that 40 percent of respondents felt their working lives were "very or extremely stressful," 26 percent felt "often or very often burned out by their work," 29 percent said they were "quite a bit or extremely stressed at work." Meanwhile, a whopping 77 percent said they experience "physical symptoms caused by stress," 73 percent regularly experience "psychological symptoms caused by stress," and a quarter of them said their work was the "number one stressor" in their lives. Ultimately, they cited a figure first reported by the World Health Organization in 2012 that said American industries cough up a whopping $300 billion annually for "health care and missed work days" as a direct result of "workplace stress." The researchers estimate that a million workers miss work every day due to stress.

The Ultimate Metabolism Killer

If for nothing else, I'd urge you to find solace in the fact that you're not the only one who's letting the pressures of work get to you. It's no wonder that we spend an estimated $14 billion on stress-relief products a year, from books to elixirs to those expensive, subscription-model meditation apps on your phone.

The truth is that your stress—much like the sugar in your diet—is something of a necessary evil in this world. If you were able to eradicate it completely from your life, you'd be even worse off. This is what scientists call the "stress paradox." In the right amounts, stress is a wonderful thing—the reason you can meet those tough deadlines, the reason you can step up to the podium in a packed house even with a crippling fear of public speaking,

THE BIGGEST WORKPLACE STRESSORS IN AMERICA

THE BIGGEST STRESSORS AT WORK

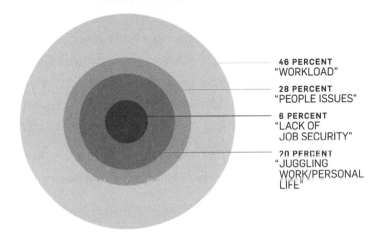

46 PERCENT
"WORKLOAD"

28 PERCENT
"PEOPLE ISSUES"

6 PERCENT
"LACK OF
JOB SECURITY"

20 PERCENT
"JUGGLING
WORK/PERSONAL
LIFE"

SYMPTOMS CAUSED BY WORK-RELATED STRESS

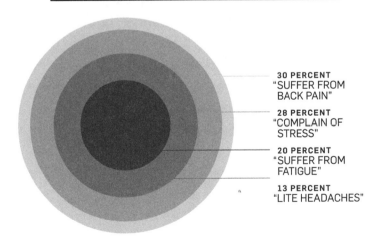

30 PERCENT
"SUFFER FROM
BACK PAIN"

28 PERCENT
"COMPLAIN OF
STRESS"

20 PERCENT
"SUFFER FROM
FATIGUE"

13 PERCENT
"LITE HEADACHES"

the reason you can leap out the window with the agility of Simone Biles if you think there's a burglar creeping inside your house—and even the reason you can build muscle at the gym. (After all, when you head to Crunch to bang out some squats, you're applying "stress" to your muscles, which will grow back stronger.)

But when you're feeling overwhelmed by your stress and you allow it to run rampant, the effect on your body is nothing short of disastrous. "Stress in and of itself can literally shut down your metabolism," says Jeffrey A. Morrison, MD, CNS, an expert in integrative medicine and metabolism issues. "It is tremendously metabolically draining. Remember: Your thyroid is the ignition switch for your metabolism."

When you're feeling heightened levels of stress, your body responds by releasing the stress hormones cortisol, adrenaline, and norepinephrine into your bloodstream. Your heart starts racing—pumping more blood—and your metabolism actually kicks into high gear. After all, the thinking goes, this is an evolutionary adaptation in place so our ancestors could run away from a prowling saber-toothed tiger. This is all very normal, if it occurs in fairly sporadic intervals. In science terms, that's called "acute" stress. When you are, like a lot of Americans, suffering from chronic stress—or repeated exposure to such situations—things start going terribly wrong with your body. According to Canada's Centre for Studies on Human Stress, chronic stress is a big factor in heart disease, high cholesterol, type 2 diabetes, and depression.

Oh, and if you're depressed? Well, you're at a 58 percent greater chance of becoming obese.

In effect, stress targets your metabolism like a cruise missile.

A 2015 study of fifty-eight women (many of whom suffered from depression in the past) published in the journal *Biological Psychiatry* explored "how stress and depression alter metabolic responses to high-fat meals in ways that promote obesity." Measuring everything from insulin to glucose to cortisol levels—as well as your resting metabolism and "fat and carbohydrate oxidation"—the researchers found that respondents who had experienced "prior day stressors" were at a serious metabolic disadvantage than the respondents who had zero stressors. In fact, they calculated that being more stressed out over the span of six hours adds up to a difference in "104 kCal." Allow me to translate that for you: Getting really stressed out can potentially amount to nearly eleven pounds of extra weight added over the course of a year. According to the study: "Higher cortisol fosters increased intake of calorie-dense 'comfort foods,' and insulin secretion rises as cortisol increases."

In a four-year British study whose findings were published last year in the journal *Obesity,* researchers measured the cortisol levels contained in locks of hair they'd plucked from 2,527 men and women over the age of fifty-four. They also tracked the subjects' "weight, body mass index, and waist circumference." Ultimately, they discovered a direct correlation between chronic stress and all three of those obesity-related factors. "People tend to report overeating and 'comfort eating' foods high in fat, sugar, and calories in times of stress," the report stated. "And the stress hormone cortisol plays an important role in metabolism and determining where fat is stored."

Meanwhile, another study, published in 2016 in the journal *Current Opinion in Behavioral Sciences,* made an equally stunning case for a straight-line connection between your metabolism and your body's stress response. "Chronic stress can lead to dietary over-consumption, increased visceral adiposity, and weight gain," the researchers, from the Institute of Neuroscience and Physiology at the Sahlgrenska Academy at the University of Gothenburg, in Sweden, write in the report.

With the tools in this book—including the Super Metabolism Movement Plan and the 10 Most Effective Non-Exercise Stress Busters, which you'll find on page 135—you'll find yourself walking through the world happier and healthier. At the end of the day, managing your stress levels is one of the surest keys for unlocking the powers of your metabolism once and for all.

SPECIAL REPORT

LIVE CLEAN, EAT CLEAN—CHEMICAL-FREE!

Why processed foods—even if they look healthy—aren't the answer. Also: why you need to look hard at many of the things that populate your home.

AS A LONG-TIME editor of health and fitness magazines—and one of the world's most enthusiastic proponents of living a smart, active, and healthy lifestyle—I've built my career on being a one-man political opposition force against a single piece of furniture: the couch.

I can't tell you how many times I've written or approved of a headline with some variation of "don't be a couch potato" or "get your butt off the couch." I've even debated with my friends on whether or not we'd be better off without them entirely. It sounds silly, until you consider that we'd all spend a lot less money, lie around less, watch less TV, and get to bed earlier. (But as a sports fan, even I know this is all wishful thinking.)

But, by 2018, little did I know how truly insidious your couch actually is—and it's got nothing to do with the gravitational pull of those lush cushions on your lazier instincts. Rather, it's got everything to do with those lush cushions.

TEN MOST EFFECTIVE NON-EXERCISE STRESS BUSTERS

For the days you don't have time to hit the gym.

Doctors tend to agree that exercise is one of the best forms of medicine out there: A boost of endorphins leaves us a calm kind of energized, a "runner's high" boosts our moods, and a habit of movement can keep debilitating diseases like depression and anxiety at bay. But sometimes, we simply don't have time to sweat. Fortunately, there are other ways to beat everyday stressors—and stay even-keeled no matter what life throws at you. Start with these ten stay-calm techniques.

MEDITATE

Why It's Effective: Chilling out has a direct impact on stress. Research out of Georgetown University Medical Center finds that after an eight-week course in mindful meditation, people with anxiety disorders lowered inflammatory markers and stress hormones in their blood by 15 percent.
How to Do It Right: You don't need to be solo in a studio with your legs crossed to meditate (though that certainly works). Meditation is about being present, focusing on your breath, and calming the mind by allowing thoughts to pass without judgment. Can't do that on your own? No biggie. Download an app like Calm or Headspace, which will walk you through guided meditations, working to improve your breathing and, in turn, bring your cortisol levels back to normal.

SIT UP STRAIGHT

Why It's Effective: Research published in the journal *Health Psychology* finds that—compared to a hunched-over position—sitting upright in the face of stress can boost self-esteem, fending off further angst. The idea boils down to something called embodied cognition, an idea that our bodies impact our emotions (and vice versa). And it could be that simply feeling taller boosts confidence, shooing stress away, researchers say.
How to Do It Right: Plant both feet on the ground, look straight ahead, straighten your back while sitting tall, and feel your shoulder blades pull back and down.

BREATHE THE RIGHT WAY

Why It's Effective: There's a reason docs sometimes prescribe breathing exercises to people struggling with truly stressful times. Deep breathing—which encourages the full exchange of oxygen in the body—activates your body's calming parasympathetic response, lowering levels of inflammatory compounds linked to stress.

How to Do It Right: Most of us breathe all wrong. Take a deep breath. If your shoulders rise on your inhale, it's time to reassess. Try again. This time, on the inhale, push your belly out. When you exhale, contract in. Your belly should rise when you breathe in and shrink when you breathe out. Take a few deep breaths with a hand on your stomach to make sure you're doing it right.

SEEK OUT NATURE (AND SUNSHINE)

Why It's Effective: A ninety-minute walk in the park can calm the mind, lowering activity in a brain region linked to depression, finds Stanford University researchers. It's not just the walking, either: People strolling through urban settings filled with traffic instead of trees didn't reap the benefits. Our bodies were designed to be in and near green spaces, forests, or the ocean, researchers say. Thus, studies confirm that these spaces are inherently relaxing.

How to Do It Right: Take your lunch break to the park near your office. Walk that tree-lined street in your neighborhood. Take your evening run off of busy main roads. Can't get outside? Some research suggests that even looking at photographs of nature can calm stressed minds. (Hello, new desktop background.)

SAY THANK YOU

Why It's Effective: Scientists are no strangers to the powers of gratitude. In fact, gratitude is linked to 23 percent lower levels of the stress hormone cortisol. Even more: A study out of the University of California, San Diego's School of Medicine found that grateful folks were happier, slept better, had more energy, and had lower levels of inflammatory biomarkers—some of which correlated with heart health.

How to Do It Right: Keep a gratitude journal. At the end of every day, write down three things you're thankful for. Some research finds that reflecting on the good at day's end can work to improve health (and sink stress).

SLEEP IT OFF

Why It's Effective: While you snooze, your brain processes all of the emotions and happenings from the day—helping your mind remain even-keeled and keeping stress levels from boiling up. That's why a lack of shut-eye can impair your ability to control your emotions, including anxiety and stress.

How to Do It Right: Simply can't log your eight to nine hours in the sack? A nap can help. A study from the Endocrine Society found that just thirty minutes of shut-eye can work to reverse the damage of a terrible night's rest—and help relieve stress, too.

PHONE A FRIEND

Why It's Effective: The healthiest (and calmest) among us tend to have something in common: a huge social life. Because friends and family can help us talk through and manage life's stressors, a strong support system is often linked with being more resilient in the face of stress itself.

How to Do It Right: Focus on quality rather than quantity. One study in the journal *Developmental Psychology* found that simply being around one close friend can decrease cortisol levels. That could be one of the reasons married people tend to have lower levels of the stress hormone cortisol.

STOP THE SNOWBALL EFFECT

Why It's Effective: Dwelling or ruminating over things that have happened or things that may happen is dangerous. Research published in the journal *PLOS One* finds that brooding over negative events is the no. 1 biggest predictor of issues like depression and anxiety and plays a huge role in how much stress you experience.

How to Do It Right: Instead of stewing over all of the ways life could go wrong, ask yourself: Is there anything in my control that I can change about this situation? If there are things you can change, change them; otherwise, try to accept the present scenario without projecting into the future—a habit that can further a spiral of negativity.

HAVE SEX

Why It's Effective: Sex often comes with a chemical cocktail of hormones like "feel good" oxytocin as well as a release of endorphins. When running through the bloodstream, these molecules can help us chill out.

How to Do It Right: Research has shown that having sex with someone else is often linked to a drop in stress levels, while masturbation is not. One study in particular found that intercourse lowered systolic blood pressure. How's that for a prescription?

EAT YOUR GREENS

Why It's Effective: Comfort foods aren't so comforting. It's the vitamins, minerals, and antioxidants in healthy eats that lower your stress levels. Take a study from the University of Otago—it found that students who ate more fruits and vegetables also tended to feel calmer and happier.

How to Do It Right: For the most bang for your (mood) buck, aim for a variety of different-colored produce—so that you're getting a variety of different nutrients. Think: a smoothie with kale or spinach, blueberries, raspberries, and bananas.

Your couch is all but guaranteed to contain flame retardant, which could be silently damaging your body. And not just a *little* bit of flame retardant, either. Chances are, it is laced with upward of two pounds of it. As the *Chicago Tribune* noted in its massive, eye-opening investigation into the rise of flame retardants in our lives, in 2012, "the amount of flame retardants in a typical American home isn't measured in parts per billion or parts per million. It's measured in *ounces and pounds*." Blood levels of flame retardants in humans have risen astronomically since the 1970s.

It will be in your couch's foam cushions and your bed pillows. It will be in carpeting, drapes, and other textiles. Though research has shown that it's largely ineffective in the event of an actual fire, the chemical industry has been hugely successful over the last few decades in making them a permanent fixture in our daily lives. According to the most recent figures by the market research firm The Freedonia Group, the global demand for flame retardants is projected to continue its sharp rise through 2018, eventually reaching 2.8 million metric tons—which translates to a value of roughly $7 billion.

Let's be clear: This is no fringe matter to simply brush off.

According to the Endocrine Society, flame retardants are just one of several endocrine-disrupting chemicals (or EDCs) that could be harming your body. In the case of Firemaster 550, a near-ubiquitous fire retardant, studies of rats show that it's an obesogenic—a chemical that causes weight gain by altering your thyroid hormone levels. Oh, and those rats they tested? They were also pregnant, and the study showed that Firemaster 550 affected the thyroid hormone levels in their offspring, as well, which grew up obese—with natural insulin resistance—and showed signs of heart disease. The effects on the children is especially chilling, because flame retardants are regular fixture in household dust that accumulates like snow across your floors, and young children are more often exposed to the chemicals than you are. In 2014, the World Health Organization and the United

Nations concluded: "Exposure to E.D.C.'s during fetal development and puberty plays a role in the increased incidences of reproductive diseases, endocrine-related cancers, behavioral and learning problems, including A.D.H.D., infections, asthma, and perhaps obesity and diabetes in humans."

Now, given that those remarks—and the aforementioned story in the *Chicago Tribune*—were from a few years back, you'd think that Firemaster 550 would've been phased out by now. Well, it's not, and the eye-opening accounts about its harmful effects, especially on children, continue to emerge. A study published in 2017 by *PLOS One* found that "exposure to FM550 . . . increased lipid accumulation, as well as the mRNA and protein levels of terminal differentiation markers in preadipocytes." For the record: Adipocytes are fat-storing cells, and lipids are fats.

Flame retardants are just one of the chemicals that are being used in abundance. EDCs are also commonly found in plastics, certain types of fruits and vegetables, and electronics. In addition to flame retardants, here are some of the most widespread and insidious:

ORGANOPHOSPHATE PESTICIDES: These are chemicals used to poison insects (as well as other animals, such as birds), which are found in agriculture and homes and gardens. According to the EPA (Environmental Protection Agency), "long-term effects have occurred following acute and often massive exposures. Symptoms that are consistently reported from exposed persons include depression, memory and concentration problems, irritability, persistent headaches and motor weakness. . . . Some of the most commonly reported early symptoms include headache, nausea, dizziness and hypersecretion, the latter of which is manifested by sweating, salivation, lacrimation and rhinorrhea. Muscle twitching, weakness, tremor, incoordination, vomiting, abdominal cramps and diarrhea all signal worsening of the poisoned state."

LEAD: According to the EPA, "Lead and lead compounds have been used in a wide variety of products found in and around our homes, including paint, ceramics, pipes and plumbing materials, solders, gasoline, batteries, ammunition, and cosmetics." It can also be found in certain drinking water, as was the case in Flint, Michigan, in 2014, when residents were given untreated water. In children, the health effects include learning problems and behavioral issues, anemia, and slowed growth. In adults it can lead to increased blood pressure, decreased kidney function, and reproductive issues.

PHTHALATES: These are chemicals used to make plastic and vinyl more flexible and soft. They're found in countless household products, from cosmetics (nail polish, shampoo, hairspray) to the plastic baggies and wraps you put your food in. Though the long-term effects on humans are unknown, they've been officially banned in baby products—such as pacifiers—since 1999.

When EDCs find their way into your bloodstream, they send your body's endocrine system into disarray. These chemicals can mimic certain hormones, camouflage the receptors, block its access to receptors, and even cause too many or too little hormones to be produced.

A study conducted by the UK's University of Reading and published in *Current Obesity Reports* in 2017 found that continuous exposure to bisphenol A—also known as BPA, a widespread chemical that's banned in baby water bottles but is commonly used to make plastics and the lining of soda cans and is often found in processed foods—is not only responsible for weight gain but also "might offer an explanation as to why obesity is an underlying risk factor for so many diseases, including cancer." Another study, published in the *Journal of Endocrinological Investigation* in 2016, found that avoiding BPA exposure is a great way to avoid disease down the road. The researchers also stated that BPA is a "serious problem of global proportion and economic and social emergencies, such as obesity, metabolic syndrome, and diabetes."

In 2016, a study published in *The Open Biotechnology Journal* went even further, saying that the explosive rise in diabetes over the last few decades can't be attributed to poor diet and lack of exercise alone. "The role of environmental chemicals exposure by the diet and their association to metabolic disorders are aspects that need to be considered and studied," the researchers, from Yale University and Italy's National Institute of Biostructures and Biosystems, wrote. Not only do chemicals like BPA likely destroy your metabolism—by interfering with insulin production and glucose oxidation—but they also may affect your central nervous system.

So, what does this mean for you?

Obviously, you can't go live in a cave, and you can't live your life in paranoia. Besides, who would even want to?

What you can do is take steps to be sure you're buying the right in-home products, such as rugs, furniture, flooring, paints, and wallpapers, and reducing your exposure to certain pesticides by eating whole fruits and vegetables and less processed foods that come prepackaged to stay fresh for outsize periods of time. You can eat less mercury in your seafood. You can buy a couch that isn't weighed down with two full pounds of flame retardant.

I know this is difficult, but a little bit here goes a long way.

Chapter 9

THE *SUPER METABOLISM MEALS*

Super Easy At-Home and On-the-Go Meals Designed to Keep Your Fat Burning All Day Long!

CONGRATULATIONS, HERO! You've made it. At long last, you've reached the end of your training. By now you've got Batman's brains and Wonder Woman's steely resolve, and you are officially ready to go fight to get the body of your dreams. But best of all? It's not even much of a fight. To win, all you really need to do is show up. And all it takes is for you to eat the right delicious foods and you'll find that you've ignited your metabolism and it will do all of the hard work for you.

Not only will you be feeling happier and more energetic, but you'll be seeing results in your body in as soon as two weeks. You'll also be making a down payment on your future health, as you'll be drastically reducing your risk of heart disease, diabetes, stroke, and cancer. Once you start boosting your intake of Super Proteins, you'll be feeding your muscles directly and burning more energy at the same time. With the right Super Fats, you'll be bulletproofing your heart while erecting a bulletproof wall between your body and excess hunger. With Super Carbs, you'll be feeding your metabolism directly with all of the right energy in the right amounts and keeping your blood-sugar levels well in control. With all of those forces combined, you'll find that your hormones will come into balance—and you'll be feeding your muscles directly—and your metabolism will quickly come back online.

In the ensuing pages, you'll find wonderfully delicious, science-backed recipes that are designed to get your metabolism burning hotter than ever. Remember, whether you're eating any of these dishes—or ordering food in a restaurant—always make sure you're getting enough of the key ingredients in this book. And once your two-day IGNITE phase is over, you'll move to . . .

THE AFTER BURN!

This is when you take the guidelines and principles contained in this book and apply them for the rest of your life, with one small twist: You can reintroduce a second cheat meal, and two to three alcoholic beverages (including beer and mixed drinks, which are strictly verboten during the IGNITE phase), back into your routine, every single week. If you're disciplined about the Super Metabolism Diet, you'll find that you'll be eating a healthy, metabolism-boosting diet and be able to treat yourself at the same time.

And here's a dirty little secret: If your life momentarily gets more difficult, your good eating habits fall by the wayside, and your stress levels rise while your sleep gets dinged, don't worry! You can always REIGNITE the Super Metabolism Diet and get your superpower back. Remember: It takes only two weeks.

BREAKFAST

QUICHE "MUFFINS" BY THE DOZEN

Make a dozen of these grab-and-go egg cups at a time and keep the extras in the refrigerator or freezer. Reheat in a toaster oven or microwave.

YOU'LL NEED

2	slices nitrite- and sugar-free bacon or ham, cut up
3	cups chopped fresh spinach
½	cup chopped tomato
2	green onions (scallions), chopped
8	large eggs
2	tablespoons unsweetened almond milk, milk, or water
¼	teaspoon dried red pepper flakes
3	tablespoons shredded Parmesan cheese (optional)

HOW TO MAKE IT

1. Preheat the oven to 325°F. Place liners in twelve muffin cups.

2. In a large skillet cook bacon until almost crisp. Add the spinach, tomato, and green onions and cook for about 1 minute to wilt the spinach. Remove from the heat.

3. In a large bowl, whisk together the eggs, milk, red pepper flakes, and, if using, the cheese. Stir in the bacon-vegetable mixture. Ladle into the prepared muffin cups.

4. Bake for 15 to 18 minutes or until the eggs are set.

Makes 12 quiche muffins.

■ **Per muffin:** 59 calories, 4 g fat (1 g saturated), 80 mg sodium, 0 g fiber, 0 g sugar, 5 g protein (calculated using unsweetened almond milk and no optional Parmesan cheese)

SERVING SUGGESTION:
Mixed berries with chopped toasted pecans.

BREAKFAST

5-MINUTE SALMON AND ARTICHOKE OMELET

Cooking salmon for dinner? Make a little extra for this protein-rich omelet that takes minutes to make and will keep you full until lunch.

YOU'LL NEED

2 teaspoons olive oil

2 or 3 large eggs, lightly beaten

½ teaspoon chopped dill

Pinch of salt

2 ounces cooked salmon, chopped (about ½ cup)

¼ cup chopped artichoke hearts packed in water or marinade, drained

1 to 2 tablespoons feta cheese crumbles

HOW TO MAKE IT

1. Heat the olive oil in a small nonstick skillet over medium heat. Add the eggs, dill, and salt and cook, using a spatula to stir and then lift the cooked egg on the bottom to let raw egg slide under.

2. When the eggs have all but set, add the salmon, artichoke hearts, and feta to one-half of the omelet. Fold the other half of the omelet over the filling and transfer to a plate.

Makes 1 serving.

■ 447 calories, 26 g fat (8 g saturated), 656 mg sodium, 2 g fiber, 2 g sugar, 23 g protein (calculated with 3 eggs; 1 tablespoon feta cheese)

BREAKFAST

CHOCO-CHIA SMOOTHIE

As well as adding protein, the avocado makes this thick and creamy. For a flavor variation, add ¼ to ½ teaspoon powdered coffee, such as Starbucks Via Instant.

YOU'LL NEED

⅓ cup unsweetened coconut milk or coconut water

1 banana

½ avocado

1 tablespoon unsweetened cacao powder

1 tablespoon almond butter or peanut butter

1 to 3 teaspoons chia seeds

¼ teaspoon vanilla extract

8 to 10 ice cubes

HOW TO MAKE IT

1. Add the coconut milk, banana, avocado, cacao, almond butter, chia seeds, and vanilla to the bowl of a blender. Add the ice.

2. Cover and blend until smooth.

Makes 1 serving.

TIP: One tablespoon of chia seeds, the ancient seeds of the Aztecs and Mayans, offers 2 grams protein and 4 grams fiber and is high in omega-3 fatty acids (supports cardiovascular function). Start with 1 teaspoon and work your way to 3 (1 tablespoon) since too much too quickly can cause digestive discomfort in some people.

■ 369 calories, 23 g fat (4 g saturated), 80 mg sodium, 14 g fiber, 18 g sugar, 9 g protein (calculated using almond butter; 1 teaspoon chia seeds)

BREAKFAST

JERKED SWEET POTATO SCRAMBLE

If your mornings are already a scramble, cook the sweet potato mixture the night before and stash it in the fridge.

YOU'LL NEED

1   medium sweet potato, skinned and finely diced

2   tablespoons lime juice

½ to 1 teaspoon finely chopped chile pepper such as scotch bonnet or jalapeño

½   teaspoon allspice

½   teaspoon salt

2   teaspoons olive oil

8   large eggs, lightly beaten

Fresh mango salsa (optional)

HOW TO MAKE IT

1. Toss the sweet potato with the lime juice, chile pepper, allspice, and ¼ teaspoon salt.

2. In a large nonstick skillet, heat the olive oil over medium-high heat. Add the potato mixture and cook for 5 to 7 minutes or until tender, stirring frequently. Remove the mixture from the skillet.

3. Add the eggs and remaining ¼ teaspoon salt to the skillet. Cook 1 minute more, then stir to scramble the eggs, cooking 2 to 3 minutes more or until cooked through but still glossy. Top with the sweet potato mixture. If desired, serve with mango salsa.

Makes 4 servings.

■ 191 calories, 12 g fat (4 g saturated), 437 mg sodium, 1 g fiber, 2 g sugar, 13 g protein (calculated with optional mango salsa)

BREAKFAST

BUENOS DÍAS BLACK BEANS

YOU'LL NEED

1¼ cups cooked or canned black beans, drained and rinsed

1 radish, halved and sliced

1 lime wedge

Pinch of chili powder

½ avocado, sliced

2 tablespoons fresh salsa

1 tablespoon Cashew Cream or plain Greek yogurt

1 tablespoon raw or toasted pumpkin seeds (optional)

HOW TO MAKE IT

1. Place the beans (hot or cold) and radish in a bowl and toss with a squeeze of lime and the chili powder. Add the avocado and fresh salsa.

2. Drizzle with the cashew cream or dollop with yogurt. If desired, sprinkle with pumpkin seeds.

Makes 1 serving.

CASHEW CREAM: Soak 1 cup raw cashews in about 4 cups water for 4 to 12 hours; drain. Place the cashews, ¼ cup fresh water, and a pinch of salt in the bowl of a strong blender. If desired, add a squeeze of lemon. Cover and blend until smooth, adding additional water if needed until the desired consistency is reached. Store in the refrigerator for up to 4 days or freeze up to 1 month. Stir before using.

■ **Cashew Cream:** 640 calories, 48 g fat (8 g saturated), 162 mg sodium, 4 g fiber, 8 g sugar, 20 g sugar

■ **Buenos Días Black Beans and Cashew Cream:** 563 calories, 24 g fat (4 g saturated), 56 mg sodium, 25 g fiber, 3 g sugar, 25 g protein (calculated without optional pumpkin seeds)

BREAKFAST

HASH IT OUT

So worth a little a.m. shredding, this hash is ultra flexible. You can sub sausage or ham for the bison or go meatless. Add chopped hot or sweet peppers or sliced mushrooms. Before serving, sprinkle on a little shredded cheddar or crushed flaxseed. Hash also makes tasty leftovers, heated up in a skillet or the oven.

YOU'LL NEED

1   pound Yukon gold potatoes, peeled and halved lengthwise (about 2 medium)

1   medium onion, quartered

1   medium carrot, peeled

1   medium cooked beet, peeled

½   pound cooked ground bison or grass-fed ground beef, crumbled

½   teaspoon salt

¼ to ½ teaspoon dried red pepper flakes or 2 teaspoons chili powder

2 to 3 tablespoons olive oil

4   large poached eggs (optional)

HOW TO MAKE IT

1. Shred the potatoes, onion, and carrot in a food processor with a grater attachment. Place in a bowl of ice water for a few minutes. Rinse in a colander until the water runs clear. Drain well and pat dry with paper towels.

2. Shred the beet in the food processor. In a large bowl, combine the potato mixture, meat, beets, salt, and red pepper flakes.

3. In a large nonstick skillet with sloping sides, heat 2 tablespoons olive oil over medium-high heat. Add the potato mixture, pressing it into the pan to make a large patty. Reduce the heat to medium and cook about 12 minutes or until the bottom of the potato mixture is golden and crisp. With a spatula gently turn large pieces of the potato mixture over, adding more oil as needed. Cook for 6 to 8 minutes more or until the bottom is golden brown. If desired, serve with poached eggs.

Makes 4 servings.

TIP: When roasting or boiling beets, cook a few extra for recipes like this one or salads. Or, finely shred a peeled raw beet for this hash. It will just be a little more crunchy.

■ **TO POACH EGGS:** Add 4 cups water and 1 tablespoon vinegar to a large skillet and bring to boiling. Reduce the heat to a simmer. Break an egg into a cup and gently add them to the water. Repeat with 3 more eggs, keeping each separate. Simmer, uncovered, for 3 to 5 minutes or until the whites are set and the yolk is a desired doneness.

■ **COMBINED:** 294 calories, 14 g fat (4 g saturated), 412 mg sodium, 4 g fiber, 4 g sugar, 20 g protein

BREAKFAST

LOADED BREAKFAST SAUSAGES

Pump up your a.m. sausages with lean turkey and a couple of veggies and feel good instead of guilty. Keep any extras in the refrigerator for up to four days or the freezer for up to six months.

YOU'LL NEED

¾   cup shredded zucchini

8   ounces ground turkey

8   ounces ground pork

¾   cup chopped mushrooms

2   cloves garlic, minced

1   tablespoon chopped fresh sage or 1 teaspoon dried sage

¼ to ½ teaspoon salt

½   teaspoon ground black pepper

HOW TO MAKE IT

1. Pat the zucchini dry with paper towels. In a large bowl, mix together the zucchini, turkey, pork, mushrooms, garlic, sage, salt, and pepper.

2. Shape the meat mixture into eight patties, about 3 inches each.

3. In a large skillet, cook the sausages, four at a time, for 8 to 10 minutes until browned (165°F internal temperature), flipping halfway through.

Makes 8 sausages.

■ 137 calories, 8 g fat (3 g saturated), 184 mg sodium, 0 g fiber, 0 g sugar, 13 g protein (calculated using ½ teaspoon salt)

BREAKFAST

PACK-AND-GO GREEN TEA YOGURT CUPS WITH SEED "GRANOLA"

Popular for its antioxidant load, Japanese matcha is made by grinding green tea leaves into a powder. Whisk it with hot water for a beverage or add it to recipes.

YOU'LL NEED

1 cup unsweetened coconut milk yogurt or Greek yogurt

1 teaspoon matcha or grated fresh ginger

¼ to ½ teaspoon ground turmeric

¼ teaspoon vanilla extract

½ cup fresh berries, such as blueberries, raspberries, or sliced strawberries, and/or pomegranate seeds

1 tablespoon chopped nuts

½ to 1 teaspoon mixed seeds, such as sunflower, sesame, chia, and/or crushed flaxseed

HOW TO MAKE IT

1. In a small bowl, combine yogurt, matcha, turmeric, and vanilla.

2. In a small storage container, layer half the berries and half the yogurt mixture; top with the nuts and mixed seeds.

Makes 1 serving.

■ 218 calories, 14 g fat (8 g saturated), 190 mg sodium, 11 g fiber, 10 g sugar, 2 g protein (calculated using coconut yogurt, ¼ teaspoon ground turmeric, ½ teaspoon mixed seeds)

■ 288 calories, 11 g fat (4 g saturated), 75 mg sodium, 3 g fiber, 17 g sugar, 25 g protein (calculated using Greek yogurt, ¼ teaspoon ground turmeric, ½ teaspoon mixed seeds)

BREAKFAST

MINT CHOCOLATE OATMEAL

YOU'LL NEED

2	teaspoons chopped fresh mint
1	cup unsweetened almond milk
½	cup rolled oats
2	tablespoons unsweetened cocoa powder
½	cup raspberries

HOW TO MAKE IT

1. Blend the mint and ½ cup almond milk in the bowl of a blender until smooth.

2. Add the mixture to the remaining milk and add in the oats.

3. Cook in the microwave for 2 minutes.

4. Remove and stir in the cocoa. Top with raspberries.

Makes 1 serving.

■ 300 calories, 12 g fat (4 g saturated), 400 mg sodium, 13 g fiber, 15 g sugar, 13 g protein

BREAKFAST

SMOKED SALMON SANDWICH

This is a New York classic, minus the bagel. The end result is a sandwich you can feel good about eating every day of the week, and given that it takes about as much time to make as it does to pour a bowl of cereal, why not?

YOU'LL NEED

¼   cup whipped cream cheese

8   slices whole-wheat or 9-grain bread, toasted

2   tablespoons capers, rinsed and chopped

½   red onion, thinly sliced

2   cups mixed baby greens

1   large tomato, sliced

   Salt and black pepper to taste

8   ounces smoked salmon

HOW TO MAKE IT

1. Spread 1 tablespoon of the cream cheese on each of four slices of toast. Top each with capers, onion, greens, and a slice or two of tomato. Lightly salt the tomato, then add as much pepper as you'd like (this sandwich cries out for a lot of it). Finish by draping a few slices of smoked salmon over the tomatoes and topping with the remaining slices of toasted bread.

Makes 4 sandwiches.

■ 280 calories, 10 g fat (3 g saturated), 460 mg sodium, 13 g fiber, 2 g sugar, 17 g protein

BREAKFAST

BERRY GOOD QUINOA BREAKFAST SALAD

This is a favorite from *Zero Belly Breakfasts,* filled with more than one hundred recipes and nutrition secrets that help melt pounds all day, every day.

YOU'LL NEED

FOR THE SALAD

1	cup quinoa, cooked and cooled
¾	cup strawberries, sliced in half
½	cup raspberries
½	cup blueberries
½	cup raw almonds, finely chopped
1½	teaspoons fresh mint, finely chopped
1½	teaspoons fresh basil, finely chopped

FOR THE DRESSING

½	teaspoon orange zest
2	tablespoons fresh orange juice
1	tablespoon fresh lemon juice
1½	teaspoons fresh lime juice
1½	teaspoons honey
½	teaspoon fresh mint, finely chopped
½	teaspoon fresh basil, finely chopped

HOW TO MAKE IT

1. In a large bowl, combine all of the salad ingredients.

2. Then, in a separate bowl or jar, whisk together all of the dressing ingredients. Drizzle the desired amount over the salad mixture.

Makes 2 servings.

■ 354 calories, 11.7 g fat (1 g saturated), 6 mg sodium, 8.7 g fiber, 9.6 g sugar, 12.2 g protein

SPECIAL REPORT

SUPER METABOLISM SMOOTHIES

Although it's always good to chew your food—remember, the mere act of chewing powers your metabolism—a quick and easy smoothie is a surefire way to fill your belly with portable protein. Enjoy.

Java Buzzed

YOU'LL NEED

4	large coffee ice cubes
1	can unsweetened coconut milk
¼	cup unsweetened almond milk
½	frozen banana
1	scoop chocolate plant-based protein powder

HOW TO MAKE IT

1. For the cubes, pour the coffee into ice cube trays and freeze. Then place the cubes into the bowl of blender with the remaining ingredients. Blend until creamy.

Serves 1

■ 300 calories, 14 g fat (10 g saturated), 270 mg sodium, 13 g fiber, 20 g sugar, 20 g protein

Mexican Chocolate

YOU'LL NEED

1	cup unsweetened almond milk
3	ice cubes
½	banana
4	tablespoons unsweetened cocoa powder
1	teaspoon chili powder
1	teaspoon cinnamon
1	teaspoon flaxseed oil
1	scoop chocolate plant-based protein powder

HOW TO MAKE IT

1. Blend all of the ingredients in the bowl of a blender until smooth.

Serves 1

■ 325 calories, 15 g fat (1 g saturated), 400 mg sodium, 18 g fiber, 8 g sugar, 26 g protein

Clean and Green

YOU'LL NEED

½ cup unsweetened almond milk

1 cup baby spinach

½ frozen banana

1 teaspoon spirulina

1 scoop vanilla plant-based protein powder

HOW TO MAKE IT

1. Blend all of the ingredients in the bowl of a blender until smooth.

Serves 1

■ 245 calories, 8 g fat (1 g saturated), 170 mg sodium, 9 g fiber, 9 g sugar, 24 g protein

Sunshine in a Glass

YOU'LL NEED

¾ cup unsweetened coconut milk

½ cup yellow raspberries

2 tablespoons fresh mint

1 teaspoon flaxseed oil

1 cup ice

1 scoop vanilla plant-based protein powder

HOW TO MAKE IT

1. Blend all of the ingredients in the bowl of a blender until smooth.

Serves 1

■ 270 calories, 14 g fat (4 g saturated), 65 mg sodium, 12 g fiber, 4g sugar, 21 g protein

10 SUPER EASY OATMEAL COMBOS

■ Using your favorite milk (or just water), prepare a half cup of steel-cut oats as directed. Stir in a tablespoon of freshly ground flaxseeds as well as diced pineapple and strawberries. Serve warm.

■ After cooking a half cup of steel-cut oats in water, stir in half of a mashed banana. Top it off with a tablespoon of organic 70–85% dark chocolate chips for a healthy dose of sweetness and antioxidants.

■ CITRUS FLARE: Add a teaspoon of honey and a tablespoon of chia seeds to a half cup of your favorite cooked oats. Zest two tablespoons of orange peel on top and finish it off with a pinch of shredded coconut. Serve warm.

■ Mix in half a flattened scoop of plant-based vanilla protein powder along with a tablespoon of chia seeds, a quarter teaspoon vanilla extract, and a quarter teaspoon cinnamon into a half cup of uncooked steel-cut oats. Transfer the blended oatmeal into an airtight container like a Mason jar, and pop it in the fridge overnight for a quick and satiating breakfast the next day.

■ PROTEIN PUNCH: Blend half a mashed banana into a half cup of cooked steel-cut oats. Then, pour in a quarter cup of liquid egg whites (the equivalent of one egg's whites) and mix thoroughly. Stir a teaspoon of almond butter in for extra creaminess and a punch of protein and healthy fats.

■ CINNAMON BUN DREAMS: Whirl a teaspoon of maple syrup, a half teaspoon of cinnamon, and a quarter teaspoon of vanilla extract into a half cup of cooked oats. Sprinkle a handful of chopped pecans on top, and serve warm.

■ Melt a square of organic 70–85% dark chocolate and swirl it into a half cup of cooked oats. Then, mash up a handful of raspberries and stir it in along with a tablespoon of natural peanut butter.

■ After cooking a half cup of steel-cut oats in water or your favorite milk, scoop in two tablespoons each of cottage cheese and vanilla Greek yogurt.

■ In a small saucepan, toss in one cup of fresh blueberries along with a third cup of water. Allow it to simmer over low heat until the berries begin to dissolve. Once the blueberries become almost fully softened, remove them from the heat and stir half of the mixture into a half cup of oats. Top it off with a teaspoon of chia seeds and a light drizzle of honey.

■ Pour a third cup of your favorite milk into a half cup of uncooked steel-cut oats. Then, dollop two tablespoons of Greek vanilla yogurt. Stir in a pinch of cardamom and a quarter teaspoon of cinnamon. Top it off with a quarter cup of chopped pistachios. Transfer the mixture into a Mason jar, and store it in the fridge overnight. Enjoy the next day.

LUNCH

VINTAGE TUNA-TOMATO SALAD

Protein-packed tuna and eggs will fill you up without the usual bread. Carrots add crunch, color, and vitamins, but you can also sub in ½ cup chopped celery, cucumber, or apple.

YOU'LL NEED

1   5-ounce can tuna (such as Wild Planet Wild Albacore Tuna), drained

2   large hard-cooked eggs, peeled and chopped

1   small carrot, shredded

¼   cup organic mayonnaise (such as Wilderness or Spectrum)

1   tablespoon balsamic vinegar

½ to 1 teaspoon curry powder

2   large tomatoes (heirloom if available)

      Grains of paradise or cracked black pepper

HOW TO MAKE IT

1. In a medium bowl, stir together the tuna, eggs, carrot, mayonnaise, vinegar, and curry powder.

2. Core the tomatoes. Cut each into wedges almost to but not through the bottoms. Fan out the wedges and top with the tuna-egg salad. Season to taste with grains of paradise.

Makes 2 servings.

TIP: Read the labels when shopping for mayonnaise and opt for one with no added sugar, if possible. You can also make this with all or part Greek yogurt.

■ 431 calories, 32 g fat (7 g saturated), 617 mg sodium, 3 g fiber, 6 g sugar, 24 g protein

LUNCH

HOT-CHILLY SUPER SMOOTHIE

Want even more protein? Add a tablespoon spirulina or whey protein powder or chia seeds. For a slightly sweeter smoothie, add half of a banana.

YOU'LL NEED

½ to ⅔ cup unsweetened coconut milk or unsweetened almond milk

1   cup chopped kale leaves

½   small cucumber, cut up

½   avocado

1   nectarine or peach, pitted, or 1 cup berries

1   tablespoon lemon juice

½   inch slice ginger, peeled

⅛   teaspoon cayenne pepper

10   ice cubes

HOW TO MAKE IT

1.   Add the milk, kale, cucumber, avocado, nectarine, lemon juice, ginger, and cayenne to the bowl of a blender. Add the ice. Cover and blend until smooth.

Makes 2 servings.

■ 124 calories, 7 g fat (2 g saturated), 29 mg sodium, 5 g fiber, 6 g sugar, 4 g protein (calculated with ½ cup unsweetened coconut milk)

LUNCH

PHO-STYLE TURKEY LETTUCE WRAPS

If you have lean ground beef or bison on hand, go ahead and sub it in for the turkey.

YOU'LL NEED

3	tablespoons tamari or coconut aminos
1	tablespoon rice vinegar
1	teaspoon 5-spice powder
1	teaspoon toasted sesame oil
12	ounces ground turkey
12	ounces bagged broccoli slaw
8	napa cabbage leaves or lettuce leaves
½	cup coarsely chopped fresh Thai basil, mint, and/or cilantro leaves

HOW TO MAKE IT

1. In a small bowl, combine the tamari, rice vinegar, 5-spice powder, and sesame oil.

2. In a large nonstick skillet, cook turkey over medium-high heat until browned. Stir in the tamari mixture. Add the broccoli slaw and cook for 2 to 3 minutes or until the slaw is crisp-tender.

3. Spoon the filling onto the cabbage leaves; top with the herbs and roll up.

Makes 4 (2-wrap) servings.

■ 239 calories, 10 g fat (2 g saturated), 362 mg sodium, 3 g fiber, 7 g sugar, 26 g protein

LUNCH

ARUGULA WITH ASPARAGUS BUNDLES AND WHIRLED MANGO

YOU'LL NEED

2   thin slices organic deli ham
     Dijon mustard
4   cooked asparagus spears or raw seedless cucumber spears
2   cups arugula
½   cup raspberries or halved and pitted cherries
2 to 3 tablespoons Whirled Mango Dressing

HOW TO MAKE IT

1. Spread the ham slices with a thin layer of mustard and cut each slice in half. Wrap a half-slice of ham around each asparagus spear, wrapping from the bottom almost to the top. Arrange the arugula on a plate and top with the wrapped asparagus spears and raspberries.

2. Drizzle with some of the Whirled Mango Dressing.

Makes 1 serving.

WHIRLED MANGO DRESSING: In the bowl of a blender, combine 1 cup diced mango, ¼ cup Greek yogurt, and 1 tablespoon apple cider vinegar. Cover and blend until smooth. Add 1 tablespoon chopped fresh mint and blend until mixed. Cover and refrigerate extra dressing for up to 1 week.

■ **COMBINED:** 149 calories, 3 g fat (1 g saturated), 730 mg sodium, 7 g fiber, 11 g sugar, 14 g protein (calculated with 2 tablespoons—half a recipe—mango dressing)

LUNCH

CHICKS AND STICKS CHOPPED SALAD

Make this salad your way. Sub in bottled vinaigrette (about ⅓ cup), swap chopped kale for the greens, or up the protein with a sprinkle of feta crumbles, diced smoked Gouda, chopped nuts, and/or avocado.

YOU'LL NEED

1   lemon

3   tablespoons olive oil

1   teaspoon Dijon or whole-grain mustard

1   9-ounce bag romaine or a crunchy lettuce blend, coarsely chopped

1   15-ounce can garbanzo beans (chickpeas), drained and rinsed

2   cups shredded cooked chicken

3   cups matchstick vegetables (such as sweet peppers, carrots, cucumber, radish, green onions [scallions], and/or zucchini cut into matchstick-size strips or chopped)

¼   cup chopped dried tomatoes (oil pack), drained, or quartered kalamata olives

HOW TO MAKE IT

1. Zest and juice the lemon. In a jar with a lid, combine the lemon juice, ½ teaspoon of the lemon zest, the olive oil, and the mustard. Cover and shake.

2. In a large bowl, layer the lettuce, beans, chicken, matchstick vegetables, and tomatoes. Toss with the dressing.

Makes 4 servings.

TIP: Leftover cooked skinless chicken or rotisserie chicken, shredded with two forks, works well.

NOTE: If toting lunch, place one serving in a storage container. Pack in a mini cooler with an ice pack or refrigerate for up to 6 hours. To make the salad up to 24 hours ahead, refrigerate the salad and dressing separately and toss before serving.

■ 282 calories, 18 g fat (3 g saturated), 366 mg sodium, 3 g fiber, 5 g sugar, 24 g protein

LUNCH

5-WAY AVOCADO BOATS

Halve and pit one avocado and top the halves with a different combo, below, for each day of the workweek.

Fruit Sundae: Mix 1 cup chopped mixed fruit with 1 teaspoon chopped fresh mint; spoon over the avocado halves. Drizzle with lime juice and sprinkle with chili powder. If desired, add a dollop of plain Greek yogurt.

- 198 calories, 11 g fat (2 g saturated), 92 mg sodium, 9 g fiber, 12 g sugar, 3 g protein

Bean Machine: Toss 1 cup cooked black beans with ¼ cup each chopped cucumber and quartered grape tomatoes. Drizzle with balsamic vinegar and top with ground black pepper or grains of paradise.

- 313 calories, 12 g fat (2 g saturated), 978 mg sodium, 17 g fiber, 2 g sugar, 16 g protein

Smashed Pea Hummus: In the bowl of a blender, combine 1 cup thawed frozen peas, 1 tablespoon olive oil, 1 tablespoon lemon juice, and 1 teaspoon fresh basil. Blend until almost smooth. Spoon atop the avocado halves. Season with salt and pepper to taste, and if desired, sprinkle with toasted pine nuts.

- 346 calories, 25 g fat (4 g saturated), 605 mg sodium, 12 g fiber, 6 g sugar, 8 g protein

Mushroom Melts: In a small nonstick skillet, cook 2 cups sliced mushrooms, ½ teaspoon chopped fresh rosemary, and a pinch of garlic salt in 1 teaspoon hot olive oil until tender. Spoon over the avocado halves and immediately sprinkle with shredded Swiss or Parmesan cheese.

- 187 calories, 16 g fat (2 g saturated), 251 mg sodium, 7 g fiber, 3 g sugar, 6 g protein

PBAs: Stir together 1 tablespoon plain Greek yogurt, 1 teaspoon unsweetened peanut butter, ¼ teaspoon curry powder, and a pinch of salt. Top the avocado halves with mini greens and chopped apple; drizzle with the peanut butter sauce.

- 199 calories, 14 g fat (2 g saturated), 265 mg sodium, 8 g fiber, 6 g sugar, 5 g protein

LUNCH

POLLOS HERMANOS BURGER

Here, you'll combine a lean grind of meat and a hugely flavorful (but surprisingly low-calorie) spiked mayo to deliver on the promise of a truly healthy burger.

YOU'LL NEED

2   tablespoons olive oil mayonnaise

2   tablespoons chopped sun-dried tomatoes

       Juice of ½ lemon

2   cloves garlic, finely minced

1   teaspoon chopped fresh rosemary

       Salt and black pepper

1   pound lean ground chicken

4   whole-wheat or potato buns (or even English muffins), split

2   cups arugula, baby spinach, or mixed greens

HOW TO MAKE IT

1. In a mixing bowl, combine the mayonnaise, sun-dried tomatoes, lemon juice, garlic, and rosemary. Season with a pinch of salt and black pepper. Set the aioli aside.

2. Preheat a grill, grill pan, or cast-iron skillet. Combine the ground chicken with ½ teaspoon salt and ½ teaspoon black pepper and mix gently. Without overworking the meat, form into four patties until the chicken just comes together.

3. When the grill or skillet is hot (if using a skillet, add a touch of oil), add the burgers. Cook on the first side for 5 to 6 minutes, until a nice crust develops. Flip and cook for 3 to 4 minutes more, until the burgers are firm but ever so slightly yielding to the touch and cooked through. Remove the burgers. While the grill or pan is hot, toast the buns.

4. Layer the bottom buns with the arugula, top each with a burger, then slather the aioli over the top of each. Crown with the bun tops and serve.

Makes 4 burgers.

■ 335 calories, 13 g fat (3 g saturated), 375 mg sodium, 3 g fiber, 5 g sugar, 30 g protein

LUNCH

GANGSTA WRAP

Unfortunately, sandwich shops and sit-down spots alike take advantage of their reputation to cram Frisbee-size tortillas with cheese, bacon, ranch, and any other high-calorie ingredients they can find. This one has a low calorie count and generous vegetable filling.

YOU'LL NEED

12   asparagus spears, woody ends removed

2   portobello mushroom caps

1   red bell pepper, halved, seeds and stem removed

1   tablespoon olive oil

    Salt and black pepper to taste

2   tablespoon olive oil mayonnaise

1   tablespoon balsamic vinegar

1   clove garlic, minced

4   large spinach or whole-wheat tortillas or wraps

2   cups arugula, baby spinach, or mixed baby greens

¾   cup crumbled goat or feta cheese

HOW TO MAKE IT

1. Preheat a grill. Toss the asparagus, mushrooms, and bell pepper with the olive oil, plus a few pinches of salt and pepper. Place on the hottest part of the grill and cook, turning occasionally, until lightly charred and tender. The asparagus should take the least amount of time (about 5 minutes) and the peppers the most (about 10). Alternatively, you can roast the vegetables in a 450°F oven for 10 to 12 minutes. Slice the mushroom caps into thin strips. If possible, peel off the charred skin of the pepper and then slice.

2. Combine the mayonnaise, vinegar, and garlic and stir to combine thoroughly. Heat the tortillas on the grill or in the microwave for 30 seconds. Spread the balsamic mayo down the middle of each tortilla, then top with the greens and cheese. Divide the grilled vegetables among the tortillas, then roll up tightly and slice each wrap in half.

Makes 4 wraps.

■ 240 calories, 13 g fat (3.5 g saturated), 450 mg sodium, 5.3 g fiber, 6 g sugar, 13 g protein

LUNCH

SEARED TUNA WITH SHAVED FENNEL, GRAPEFRUIT, AND ARUGULA

Jason Lawless, a classically trained chef, whipped this up for my *Zero Belly Cookbook* and it's been my go-to ever since. It takes just fifteen minutes to make.

YOU'LL NEED

1	fennel bulb, thinly sliced into half-moons
3	cups packed arugula
1	large ruby red grapefruit, segmented
¼	cup coarsely chopped fresh parsley
3	tablespoons Zero Belly Vinaigrette
1	pound Seared Tuna

HOW TO MAKE IT

1. Combine the salad ingredients and vinaigrette in a large bowl. Mix well and divide among four plates.

2. Top each with 4 ounces of seared, sliced tuna.

FOR THE VINAIGRETTE

3   tablespoons raw apple cider vinegar

⅓   cup olive oil

¾   teaspoon Dijon mustard

¾   teaspoon raw Manuka honey

⅛   teaspoon kosher salt

⅛   teaspoon freshly ground black pepper

HOW TO MAKE IT

1. Combine the ingredients in a glass jar and shake vigorously until emulsified.

2. Store in the fridge for up to 2 weeks. Shake before serving. Makes ½ cup.

FOR THE SEARED TUNA

1½   teaspoons kosher salt

1½   teaspoons ground coriander

1½   teaspoons ground fennel seed

1½   teaspoons freshly ground black pepper

1   tablespoon olive oil

1   pound fresh Ahi tuna

HOW TO MAKE IT

1. Combine the salt and spices in a small bowl. Sprinkle the tuna evenly with the spice mix and set aside to let marinate for 5 minutes.

2. Place a nonstick pan over medium-high heat and add the olive oil. Once the olive oil is hot, add the tuna to the pan with a pair of tongs and let it sear, undisturbed, for 1 minute.

3. Flip the tuna over and sear for 1 minute more. Transfer the tuna to a clean plate to cool.

Serves 4.

■ 231 calories, 8 g fat (2 g saturated), 400 mg sodium 3 g fiber, 11 g sugar, 29 g protein

12 SUPER EASY BURGER COMBOS

■ Combine ground lamb with salt, pepper, and fresh or dried rosemary. Sandwich on toasted buns with garlic- and olive oil–spiked yogurt, arugula, and roasted red peppers.

■ Combine a can of black beans with half a chopped onion, a few spoonfuls of salsa, a quarter cup of breadcrumbs, the juice of one lime, and salt and pepper to taste. Whirl through a food processor. Form into patties, grill or broil, and serve on buns topped with more salsa.

■ Rub portobello caps with olive oil, salt, and pepper, and grill until soft and lightly charred.

■ Brush a turkey or beef burger with your favorite barbecue sauce a minute or two before it finishes cooking. Top with sharp Cheddar and caramelized or grilled onions (and bacon, if you really want to indulge).

■ BREAKFAST BURGER: Mix ground turkey with chunks of apple, some maple syrup, and a pinch of cinnamon. Grill or cook the patties in a skillet, then place on a toasted English muffin and crown with a fried egg.

■ Top a grilled beef burger with Swiss, a slice or two of ham, pickle slices, and a good bit of Dijon. Cook the entire burger in a cast-iron skillet, turning once, using a heavy pan to compress the burger, as if making a crispy panini.

■ Grill patties made with lean pork or chicken and glaze them with bottled teriyaki sauce as they cook. Grill slices of onion and pineapple at the same time. Combine the burgers with the onion, pineapple, sliced jalapeño, and more teriyaki on toasted buns.

■ FIESTA BURGER: Grill beef or chicken patties for 4 minutes on one side, flip, and top with a scoop of canned roasted chilies and a slice of Jack cheese. Dress with salsa and guacamole.

■ Remove a pound of chicken or turkey sausage from their casings and form into patties. Grill or broil—topping each with a slice of provolone after you flip—until cooked all the way through. Top with sautéed onions and peppers.

■ **BLACK AND BLUE:** Rub bison or beef patties with blackening spices. Cook in a cast-iron skillet and top with crumbled blue cheese and sautéed mushrooms.

■ Mix ground turkey with minced shallot, fresh thyme, and Dijon. Grill or broil the patties, adding a slice of the Brie just before they finish cooking. Place on toasted English muffins with baby mixed greens, Dijon, and thinly sliced apple.

■ Form patties using lean ground sirloin. Make a deep indentation with your thumb into each and stuff with a tablespoon of blue or goat cheese, then fold the meat over to completely cover the cheese.

DINNER

RICED CAULIFLOWER AND SHRIMP TABBOULEH

YOU'LL NEED

¾   cup boiling water

½   cup bulgur wheat

½   teaspoon salt

1   cup halved yellow and/or red grape tomatoes

¾   cup riced cauliflower

⅓   cup chopped fresh mint

½   cup chopped fresh flat-leaf parsley

¼   cup sliced green onions (scallions)

3   tablespoons olive oil

3   tablespoons lemon juice

¼   teaspoon ground black pepper

1   pound peeled and deveined cooked shrimp, halved

HOW TO MAKE IT

1. In a large bowl, pour the boiling water over the wheat and ¼ teaspoon of the salt. Let it stand at room temperature for 1 hour.

2. Stir in the tomatoes, cauliflower, mint, parsley, green onions, olive oil, and lemon juice. Season with remaining ¼ teaspoon salt and the pepper. Fold in the cooked shrimp. Cover and refrigerate for 4 to 24 hours.

Makes 4 servings.

TIP: For riced cauliflower, chop the raw cauliflower in the bowl of a food processor until the size of couscous. You can also buy cauliflower "rice" pre-riced in some markets.

■ 240 calories, 12 g fat (2 g saturated), 470 mg sodium, 2 g fiber, 1 g sugar, 38 g protein

DINNER

GRILLED CAESAR SALADS WITH AVOCADO DRESSING

YOU'LL NEED

½ small avocado

¼ cup plain Greek yogurt

1 tablespoon apple cider vinegar

½ teaspoon Dijon mustard

1 teaspoon chopped fresh tarragon or chives

1 romaine heart, halved lengthwise

½ teaspoon olive oil

1 cup chopped cooked turkey, chicken, or canned tuna

1 slice sprouted bread, toasted and cubed for croutons

HOW TO MAKE IT

1. For the dressing, in the bowl of a food processor, combine the avocado, Greek yogurt, vinegar, mustard, and tarragon. Thin with water if needed until just pourable.

2. Brush the romaine halves with olive oil and grill, cut-sides down, for 4 to 6 minutes or until slightly charred on the edges. Transfer to two dinner plates. Spoon the dressing over the romaine; top with turkey and bread croutons.

Makes 2 servings.

■ 275 calories, 11 g fat (3 g saturated), 557 mg sodium, 5 g fiber, 5 g sugar, 30 g protein (calculated with 1 cup chopped turkey)

DINNER

TANDOORI CHICKEN THIGHS (WITH ROASTED BROCCOLI)

Roasted broccoli goes well with this Indian-style chicken but so does cooked barley tossed with coconut oil and toasted cashews.

YOU'LL NEED

1   8-ounce carton plain or coconut yogurt
1   tablespoon lemon juice
1   tablespoon garam masala seasoning
1   tablespoon grated ginger
½   teaspoon garlic salt
8   small bone-in chicken thighs, skinned

HOW TO MAKE IT

1. In a bowl, combine the yogurt, lemon juice, garam masala, ginger, and garlic salt. Place the chicken in a 2-quart rectangular baking dish. Pour the marinade over the chicken. Cover and chill for 2 to 24 hours.

2. Preheat the oven to 400°F. Place the chicken on a rack in a shallow baking pan. Roast, uncovered, for 40 to 45 minutes or until no longer pink inside.

Makes 4 servings.

SIDE DISH SUGGESTION:
ROASTED BROCCOLI: Cut 1 head of broccoli into florets, discarding the woody stems. In a large bowl, toss the broccoli with 2 tablespoons olive oil and salt and lemon pepper to taste. Arrange on a foil-lined 15 x 10-inch rimmed baking sheet and roast in the same oven as the chicken for about 20 minutes, until crisp-tender and lightly browned on the edges.

■ **COMBINED:** 360 calories, 12 g fat (2 g saturated), 493 mg sodium, 1 g fiber, 2 g sugar, 57 g protein

DINNER

BISON-EDAMAME NACHOS

For a twist, make tacos or burritos with the tortillas and omit the oil or use the filling for lettuce wraps.

YOU'LL NEED

4   taco-size sprouted whole-grain tortillas (such as Ezekiel)

1   teaspoon olive oil

1¼ teaspoons chili powder

½   pound ground bison or lean grass-fed beef

¼   cup chopped onion

1   small carrot, shredded

½   teaspoon garlic salt

¾   cup frozen shelled edamame

½   cup salsa

     Desired toppings such as guacamole, shredded spinach, shredded pepper Jack cheese, and/or chopped fresh cilantro (optional)

HOW TO MAKE IT

1. Preheat the oven to 400°F. Brush the tortillas with the olive oil and ¼ teaspoon chili powder. With a scissor, cut the tortillas into wedges. Arrange on a rimmed baking sheet and bake for 8 to 10 minutes or until crisp. Transfer to a platter.

2. In a large skillet, cook the bison, onion, carrot, the remaining 1 teaspoon of the chili powder, and the garlic salt until the meat is browned. Stir in the edamame and cook for 5 minutes more. Spoon the mixture atop the tortilla chips. Serve with salsa and the desired toppings.

Makes 2 servings.

■ 488 calories, 18 g fat (5 g saturated), 1,129 mg sodium, 14 g fiber, 3 g sugar, 37 g protein (calculated without optional toppings)

DINNER

SHEET-PAN PORK (WITH ROASTED CAULIFLOWER AND ONIONS)

YOU'LL NEED

1   tablespoon olive oil

1   tablespoon whole-grain mustard

2   teaspoons chopped fresh rosemary or sage

½   teaspoon fennel seeds, crushed

¼   teaspoon garlic salt

1   pork tenderloin (1 to 1¼ pounds)

HOW TO MAKE IT

1. Preheat the oven to 425°F. In a small bowl, stir together the olive oil, mustard, rosemary, fennel seeds, and garlic salt; spread all over the pork. If desired, cover and refrigerate for up to 8 hours.

2. Place the pork on a foil-lined 15 x 10-inch rimmed baking sheet. Roast for 25 to 30 minutes or until the pork is 140°F. Let stand for 5 minutes before slicing.

Makes 4 servings.

SIDE DISH SUGGESTION:
CAULIFLOWER AND ONIONS: Cut 1 head of cauliflower into florets and 1 large sweet onion into wedges; toss with 1 tablespoon olive oil and salt and pepper to taste. Arrange the vegetables around the pork on the baking sheet and roast as directed above until the vegetables are tender and lightly browned on the edges. If desired, drizzle with a little balsamic vinegar for the last 5 minutes of the cooking time.

■ **COMBINED:** 222 calories, 11 g fat (2 g saturated), 366 mg sodium, 4 g fiber, 7 g sugar, 21 g protein

DINNER

CRISPY CHICKEN BAHN MI BOWLS

Bahn mi sandwiches are usually big on bread and long on ingredients. Check out these simplified gluten-free bowls with similar flavors. If you have lime wedges and cilantro on hand, use them to garnish the bowls. Miss the bread? Nestle everything in sprouted whole-grain tortillas.

YOU'LL NEED

1	cup thinly sliced cucumber
½	cup shredded daikon radish and/or carrot
3	tablespoons unseasoned rice vinegar
2	teaspoons tamari or coconut aminos
1	large egg, slightly beaten
	Hot sauce (with no sugar)
12	gluten-free seed crackers (such as Mary's Gone Crackers), finely crushed
2	skinless, boneless chicken breast halves, thicker sides pounded slightly to flatten
1	teaspoon coconut or olive oil
2	tablespoons organic mayonnaise

HOW TO MAKE IT

1. In a small bowl, combine the cucumber, daikon, 2 tablespoons rice vinegar, and 1 teaspoon of the tamari; set aside.

2. In a shallow bowl, combine the egg, remaining 1 teaspoon of tamari, and a dash of hot sauce. Place the crushed crackers in a large resealable plastic bag. Dip the chicken breasts in the egg mixture then in the crackers, coating them on all sides. In a large nonstick skillet, heat the coconut oil over medium heat. Add the chicken breasts and cook for 6 to 8 minutes or until no longer pink, turning halfway through.

3. Stir together the mayonnaise, remaining 1 tablespoon of rice vinegar, and hot sauce to taste.

4. Place the chicken breasts in two bowls. Using a slotted spoon, top with the vegetables. Dollop with the mayonnaise mixture.

Makes 2 servings.

■ 294 calories, 18 g fat (3 g saturated), 585 mg sodium, 1 g fiber, 3 g sugar, 28 g protein (calculated with tamari, 1 teaspoon hot sauce, and olive oil)

DINNER

HAZELNUT-CRUSTED SALMON (WITH WILTED KALE)

YOU'LL NEED

2   6-ounce salmon fillets or arctic char fillets, ¾-inch thick, skinned

2   tablespoons chopped hazelnuts, pecans, or raw pumpkin seeds

2   tablespoons coconut oil or butter, softened

2   tablespoons whole-wheat panko breadcrumbs

1   tablespoon chopped chives or tarragon

2   teaspoons grated Pecorino or Parmesan cheese

¼   teaspoon lemon pepper

HOW TO MAKE IT

1. Preheat the oven to 450°F. Place the fish on one end of a foil-lined
    15 x 10-inch rimmed baking sheet. Stir together the nuts, coconut oil,
    breadcrumbs, cheese, and lemon pepper. Spoon the nut mixture onto
    the fish and pat gently to spread.

2. Bake the fish for 6 to 8 minutes or until the fish flakes with a fork. If desired,
    serve over Wilted Kale.

Makes 2 servings.

SIDE-DISH SUGGESTION:
**WILTED KALE: Toss 4 cups baby kale with 2 teaspoons olive oil and
¼ teaspoon salt. Place on the foil-lined rimmed baking sheet next to the fish
and bake for 3 to 4 minutes or just until wilted, tossing gently halfway
through the baking time. If desired, drizzle with 2 teaspoons lemon juice.**

■ **COMBINED:** 432 calories, 25 g fat (14 g saturated), 621 mg sodium, 3 g fiber,
3 g sugar, 41 g protein

DINNER

STEAMED MUSSELS AND FENNEL

Mussels are more than restaurant food. They are quick to fix and pair here with beans for a protein-filled main dish. Want an extra boost of protein and flavor? Garnish with toasted pine nuts before serving.

YOU'LL NEED

1   fennel bulb

1   teaspoon olive oil

3   cloves garlic, thinly sliced

1   15-ounce can cannellini beans, rinsed and drained

1   cup canned diced fire-roasted tomatoes

½   cup low-sodium chicken broth or water

1   tablespoon balsamic vinegar

1   pound fresh mussels*

HOW TO MAKE IT

1. Core the fennel and cut it into wedges. Chop 1 tablespoon fennel fronds; set aside.

2. In a Dutch oven, heat the olive oil over medium heat. Add the fennel and garlic and cook for about 5 minutes or until the fennel is almost tender, stirring occasionally.

3. Stir in the beans, tomatoes, broth, and vinegar. Add the mussels. Bring to boiling. Reduce the heat. Simmer, covered, for 3 to 4 minutes or until the shells open. Discard any mussels that don't open. Sprinkle with the reserved fennel fronds.

Makes 4 servings.

TIP: Mussel Management: When buying mussels, look for ones that are tightly closed or that close tightly when tapped. Before using, scrub the mussels under water and remove any beards (stringy bits outside the shell).

■ 335 calories, 7 g fat (1 g saturated), 673 mg sodium, 7 g fiber, 5 g sugar, 34 g protein

DINNER

GRILLED SKIRT STEAK WITH OLIVE TZATZIKI

YOU'LL NEED

¼   cup lemon juice

¼   cup chopped onion

3   tablespoons olive oil

2   tablespoon chopped fresh oregano

¼   teaspoon dried red pepper flakes

¼   teaspoon salt

1½   pounds beef skirt steak or flank steak (scored)

HOW TO MAKE IT

1. For the marinade, combine the lemon juice, onion, olive oil, oregano, and red pepper flakes in a large resealable plastic bag set in a shallow dish. If making Tomato Kabobs (see next page), remove 2 tablespoons of the marinade and refrigerate until needed. Add the steak to the bag, turning to coat. Seal the bag and refrigerate for 2 to 8 hours, turning the bag occasionally.

2. Drain the steak and discard the marinade in bag. Grill the steak directly over medium heat/coals for 10 to 12 minutes, or until the internal temperature reaches 145° F (for medium-rare). Cover and let stand for 5 minutes. Thinly slice the steak diagonally across the grain. Serve with Tzatziki Sauce and, if desired, Tomato Kabobs.

TZATZIKI SAUCE: In a small strainer place ½ cup shredded cucumber. Sprinkle with salt and let stand for 5 minutes. Press the cucumber to remove any excess liquid. Transfer the cucumber to a medium bowl and stir in 1 cup plain Greek yogurt, 1 tablespoon apple cider vinegar, 1 tablespoon chopped pitted green olives, and 1 clove garlic, minced.

SERVING SUGGESTION:

TOMATO KABOBS: Brush 16 cherry tomatoes with the reserved marinade from page 182. Thread the tomatoes onto skewers* and grill next to the steak for 4 to 6 minutes until warm and starting to brown.

■ **COMBINED:** 508 calories, 30 g fat (8 g saturated), 220 mg sodium, 1 g fiber, 6 g sugar, 49 g protein

TIP: If using bamboo skewers, soak them in water for 30 minutes first to keep them from burning.

DINNER

WEEKNIGHT PENNE WITH VEGGIES AND CHICKEN SAUSAGE

YOU'LL NEED

1   8-ounce package corn-and-quinoa penne pasta or whole-wheat penne pasta
2   cups small broccoli florets
1   tablespoon olive oil
2   cups sliced mushrooms
4   links fully cooked Italian-style chicken sausage, sliced
1   large red bell pepper
½   cup chicken broth
¼   cup fresh basil, cut into strips
    Parmesan cheese (optional)

HOW TO MAKE IT

1. Cook the pasta according to package directions, adding the broccoli for the last 2 minutes. Drain in a colander and return it to the pan.

2. Meanwhile, in a large nonstick skillet, heat the olive oil over medium heat. Add the mushrooms and sausage and cook until browned. Add sweet pepper and cook 1 minute more. Add the broth and bring to boiling. Reduce the heat and cook for 5 minutes; add to the pasta-broccoli mixture. Toss gently with basil and, if desired, the cheese.

Makes 6 servings.

■ 263 calories, 8 g fat (2 g saturated), 298 mg sodium, 4 g fiber, 3 g sugar, 13 g protein (calculated without optional cheese)

DINNER

INDIAN STIR-FRY WITH BLISTERED GREEN BEANS

YOU'LL NEED

2   tablespoons coconut oil or grapeseed oil, plus more if needed

1   pound green beans, trimmed

1   medium onion, halved and sliced

2   cloves garlic, minced

1   jalapeño pepper, seeded and minced

1   tablespoon grated fresh ginger

1   tablespoon water

1   tablespoon ground coriander

1   teaspoon ground cumin

¼   teaspoon ground turmeric

1¼   pounds boneless lamb or beef sirloin steak, cut into bite-size pieces

HOW TO MAKE IT

1. In a large skillet, heat the coconut oil over medium-high heat. Add the green beans and cook, without stirring, until the beans begin to develop brown "blistered" spots. Continue to cook, tossing regularly, until the beans are crisp-tender. Remove the beans from the skillet.

2. To the same hot skillet add the onion, garlic, jalapeño, and ginger. Cook and stir for 2 minutes. In a small bowl, stir together the water, coriander, cumin, and turmeric and add to the onion mixture. Add the meat (and more oil if needed). Cook for about 8 minutes more or until the meat is cooked through, stirring frequently. Stir in the green beans and heat through.

Makes 4 servings.

SERVING SUGGESTION:
If desired, serve stir-fry over hot cooked barley or farro tossed with lime and chopped fresh cilantro.

■ 416 calories, 24 g fat (14 g saturated), 8 mg sodium, 2 g fiber, 2 g sugar, 40 g protein

DINNER

COFFEE-RUBBED STEAK

Coffee and steak might seem like an unlikely partnership, but the flavor of beef is actually heightened by the robust notes of java.

YOU'LL NEED

1½   teaspoons finely ground coffee or espresso

1½   teaspoons chili powder

     Salt and black pepper to taste

1   pound flank or skirt steak

     Spoonful of pico de gallo

1   lime, quartered

HOW TO MAKE IT

1.   Preheat a grill, grill pan, or cast-iron skillet. Combine the coffee grounds with the chili powder, plus a few generous pinches of salt and pepper. Rub the spice mixture all over the steak. Cook the beef for 3 to 4 minutes per side, depending on the thickness, until slightly firm but still yielding.

2.   Let the steak rest for at least 5 minutes, then slice thinly against the grain of the meat. Serve with a big scoop of pico de gallo and a wedge of lime.

Makes 4 servings.

■ 200 calories, 9 g fat (4 g saturated), 425 mg sodium, 0 g fiber, 2 g sugar, 24 g protein (calculated with ¼ cup pico de gallo per serving)

11 SUPER EASY CHICKEN COMBOS

■ Grind almonds in the bowl of a food processor until they're as fine as breadcrumbs. Smear chicken cutlets all over with Dijon mustard, then dip them into the almonds. Bake in a 425°F oven for about 12 minutes, until crispy on the outside and cooked all the way through.

■ Use a paring knife to cut a pocket into the side of a chicken breast. Stuff with sun-dried tomatoes, toasted pine nuts, and feta. Roast in a 450°F oven for 10 to 12 minutes, until cooked through.

■ Pound a chicken breast until uniformly ¼ inch thick. Rub with salt, pepper, and olive oil and grill until lightly charred. Top with chopped figs, goat cheese, and arugula.

■ Combine 2 tablespoons red or green curry paste with a can of light coconut milk and 1 cup chicken stock and simmer in a medium sauce pan. Stir in chunks of chicken breast, chopped bok choy, and sliced mushrooms and simmer for 10 minutes. Serve over brown rice with a wedge of lime.

■ Place a breast in the center of a large piece of aluminum foil. Top with artichoke hearts, sliced fennel, cherry tomatoes, pitted olives, and a splash of olive oil and white wine. Fold up the foil to create a sealed packet and cook in a 400°F oven for 20 minutes.

■ Combine 1 cup orange juice with ½ cup soy sauce and 1 tablespoon minced fresh ginger. Boil until thick enough to coat the back of a spoon, about 10 minutes. Grill or broil chicken breasts until cooked through, and brush with sauce after.

■ Bring 1 cup balsamic vinegar and 2 cups chicken broth to a simmer. Add chicken breasts and poach over very low heat for about 10 minutes, until cooked through. Remove the chicken breasts, raise the heat, and boil until the liquid reduces in volume by half. Spoon over the chicken.

■ Combine 2 tablespoons Dijon mustard with 1 tablespoon each of soy sauce, brown sugar, and melted butter. Brush it on the chicken before and during cooking.

■ Place bone-in, skin-on chicken breasts in a roasting pan with chunks of potato, onion, and carrot. Combine ½ cup olive oil with 3 cloves minced garlic and 1 tablespoon chopped fresh rosemary. Pour this mixture over the chicken and vegetables, season with salt and pepper, and roast in a 400°F oven for 25 minutes.

■ Soak breasts or thighs in lime juice, cumin, garlic, and some canned chipotle pepper for 1 hour. Grill until nicely charred and serve with guacamole, salsa, and hot corn tortillas.

■ Cook bone-in, skin-on chicken breasts in a skillet until crispy and cooked all the way through. Remove from the skillet. Add minced shallots and mushrooms and cook until browned. Stir in 2 parts white wine and 1 part cream and cook until slightly thickened. Pour over the chicken.

THE BEST FOOD PAIRINGS FOR WEIGHT LOSS!

Although it may sound counterintuitive, there's sound science behind my recommendations here. But before you get too excited and double up on ice cream and cookies, realize that this trick does have some caveats. If you want to trim your waist in record time, you'll need to pair the right foods together on one plate. All the mighty duos below either fry fat, beat bloat, or boost metabolism:

CAYENNE + CHICKEN

■ Turn up the heat on your belly bulge by flavoring your chicken with a dash of cayenne powder. Protein-rich foods like poultry not only boost satiety but also help people eat less at subsequent meals, according to research. But that's not all: It can also increase post-meal calorie burn by as much as 35 percent! If you thought it couldn't get much better than that, think again! Researchers say that chili pepper can also help blast away stubborn belly fat! If you ask us, there's no better reason to sprinkle some onto your chicken before it hits the grill.

BELL PEPPERS + EGGS

■ Grab a bell pepper and a few eggs and get crackin'! This mighty fat-frying duo is sure to help you fit into your skinny jeans in no time. Eggs contain a metabolism-boosting nutrient called choline, and peppers are a good source of vitamin C. What does vitamin C have to do with weight loss? Getting an adequate amount of the nutrient can help fight off cortisol, a hormone that causes fat to accumulate around the midsection. Chop some peppers, add them to a hot pan with some olive oil, add in two or three eggs, and scramble them up to stay slim.

OATMEAL + BERRIES

■ If you're trying to lose weight, oatmeal topped with berries is another delicious fat-frying breakfast option you might want to consider. What makes the duo so powerful? They each contain insoluble fiber, which, according to Canadian researchers, boosts levels of ghrelin—a hormone that controls hunger. Plus, berries are packed with chemicals called polyphenols that aid weight loss and can actually stop fat from forming. Adding this meal to your weekly repertoire is sure to help you see your six-pack before swimsuit season.

HONEYDEW + RED GRAPES

■ Fight fat and banish bloating with a fruit salad comprised of honeydew and red grapes. Melon is a natural diuretic, so it helps fight the water retention responsible for making you look puffy even though you have a toned stomach. Red grapes add fuel to the better-belly fire because they contain an antioxidant called anthocyanin that helps calm the action of fat-storage genes. This dynamic duo makes for a delicious, healthy dessert and is sure to turn your two-pack into a six-pack—stat!

PISTACHIOS + ALMONDS

■ While a snack mix comprised of cereal and pretzels may taste good, it's not going to give you that tight stomach you crave. Ditch the starchy carbs and replace them with a combination of pistachios and almonds. According to researchers, reaching for these nuts in lieu of carbohydrate-based foods can help speed the rate of weight loss. More good news: A study printed in the *Journal of the International Society of Sports Nutrition* found that the amino acid L-arginine, found in almonds, helps the body burn more fat and carbs during workouts, too. So while you're doubling down on the workouts before spring break, make sure your diet is doing double duty, too!

YOGURT + CINNAMON

■ You've almost reached your weight-loss goal, but those last few pounds seem to be holding on for dear life. Ditch the last bit of flab with a daily dose of vitamin D–fortified yogurt (we like Stonyfield Organic). A *Nutrition Journal* study found that diets rich in both calcium and vitamin D can significantly decrease the amount of fat the body absorbs and stores. Why should you add a sprinkle of cinnamon to your container, you ask? Not only does it taste great, but it also contains powerful antioxidants that improve body composition and insulin sensitivity. Animal studies have also found that consuming cinnamon can ward off the accumulation of belly chub. Enjoy this tasty duo as a quick, on-the-go breakfast or an afternoon snack.

SPINACH + AVOCADO OIL

■ If your monster appetite is making it difficult for you to trim down, consider making a sautéed side dish or salad with some avocado oil and spinach. How will eating these foods help you slim down? Avocado oil is rich in monounsaturated fats that help ward off hunger. And high-volume, low-calorie greens like spinach help fill you up without filling you out. Plus, studies show that women who eat foods with high water content, such as leafy greens, have lower BMIs and smaller waistlines than those who don't load their plates with this type of food. So eat plenty of green to get lean.

BANANAS + SPINACH

■ Slightly green bananas are rich in something called resistant starch. This type of starch not only boosts satiety but also—as the name implies— resists digestion. The result: The body has to work harder to digest the food, which promotes fat oxidation and reduces abdominal fat. What's more, bananas are rich in potassium, a nutrient that helps banish pesky bloat that can make you look less trim and fit than you actually are. Pair this mighty fruit with spinach, a low-cal veggie that boosts satiety and aids post-pump recovery, to create a fat-frying smoothie in just seconds. Simply throw a small banana, two handfuls of spinach, and a cup of organic 1% or carrageenan-free almond milk (we like Silk Unsweetened variety) into a blender with a couple of ice cubes, blend, and enjoy!

TUNA + GINGER

■ Want to look slim and fit on the beach? Look no further than the ocean—or at least the oceanside sushi joint. Pairing a tuna roll or a few pieces of tuna sashimi with ginger, the oft-overlooked pickled spice that comes on your plate, can help your abs shine through. Ginger accelerates gastric emptying, which helps diminish that "food baby" look more rapidly than other foods, and it also blocks several genes and enzymes in the body that promote bloat-causing inflammation. Tuna's role on this team is important, too; it's a primo source of docosahexaenoic acid (DHA), a type of omega-3 fatty acid that can ward off stress chemicals that promote flab storage and down-regulate fat genes in the stomach, stopping belly-fat cells from growing larger.

APPLES + WATERMELON

■ All fruits are healthy, but some fight fat better than others. And when you put the best of the best together in one simple fruit salad, you've got yourself a solid defense against health-harming flab. Apples are one of the very best sources of fiber in the fruit kingdom—and the nutrient is integral to reducing visceral fat. In fact, a recent study found that over five years, for every 10-gram increase in soluble fiber eaten per day, visceral fat diminished by 3.7 percent. Watermelon, which is one of our Best Fruits for Fat Loss, adds fuel to the waist-whittling fire by improving lipid profiles and lowering fat accumulation. This dynamic duo makes for a delicious, healthy dessert or anytime snack.

CORN + BEANS

■ While eating something that can make your belly bloated may not sound like the best way to lose weight, it's actually a solid strategy. Eating a calorie-restricted diet that includes four weekly servings of protein- and fiber-rich legumes aids weight loss more effectively than a calorie-equivalent diet that doesn't include beans, say Spanish researchers. Besides tasting delicious, pairing beans with corn can help boost the slimming effects. Corn, like bananas, contains resistant starch, a type of carb that dodges digestion. In turn, the body isn't able to absorb as many of the corn's calories or glucose, a nutrient that's stored as fat if it's not burned off, aiding weight-loss efforts. To reap the benefits, create a tasty corn and bean side dish. Combine salt- and BPA-free cans of corn and beans in a saucepan and warm over medium heat. Season with ground pepper and cilantro. Add the mixture to greens for a waist-trimming salad, use it as a flavorful topper for grilled chicken, or load the mixture into a toasted whole-grain pita pocket for a quick, on-the-go lunch.

COFFEE + CINNAMON

■ Fight fat and ward off diet-derailing hunger with a cup of cinnamon-spiked coffee. The spice is sitting in just about every coffee shop in America, but very few people sprinkle any in their cup—big mistake. Cinnamon is practically calorie-free and can add a major flavor punch to your morning java. What's more, it contains powerful antioxidants that are proven to reduce the accumulation of belly flab. Pair that with an appetite-suppressing cup of caffeine, and you've got quite the powerful six-pack-carving duo. Bonus: If you're making coffee at home, add cinnamon right into your brew pot with the grinds for an even better taste and all the same weight-loss benefits.

POTATOES + PEPPER

■ Thanks to the popularity of low-carb diets, white potatoes have been unfairly blacklisted. However, a second look at the science reveals that the spuds are actually powerful hunger tamers that can help you lose weight. In fact, Australian researchers found that potatoes are actually more filling than fiber-rich brown rice and oatmeal! The root vegetable is also a good source of bloat-banishing potassium, so it can help you look slimmer almost immediately. But just because potatoes are a go doesn't mean your favorite high-cal toppings also have the green light. We're looking at you, bacon bits! Our suggestion: Enjoy half a baked potato with a bit of olive oil and fresh pepper instead. Piperine, the powerful compound that gives black pepper its taste, may interfere with the formation of new fat cells—a reaction known as adipogenesis—which can help trim your waist, zap body fat, and lower cholesterol levels. It's a triple win!

YOGURT + RASPBERRIES

■ Ditch that layer of cold-weather chub with a slimming bowl of yogurt and berries. Consuming a combination of calcium and vitamin D—what's typically found in a tub of vitamin D–fortified yogurt—can significantly decrease belly chub and fat absorption in overweight populations, a *Nutrition Journal* study found. To get similar results at home, start your day with some Stonyfield Organic Fat-Free Plain Yogurt and top it with fiber-packed raspberries. The fruit is a great source of insoluble fiber that, according to Canadian researchers, boosts levels of ghrelin—a hormone that controls hunger. Plus, berries are packed with chemicals called polyphenols that aid weight loss and can actually stop fat from forming. Enjoy this tasty duo as a quick breakfast or afternoon snack.

GARLIC + FISH

■ Fish host long chains of omega-3 fatty acids, which help to lower triglycerides and reduce inflammation. They're also great sources of muscle-building protein, and the more muscle you have on your body, the higher your metabolic rate. Throw garlic into the mix, and you have a lethal weapon for fighting belly fat. According to a study published in the journal *Nutrition Research and Practice*, women who ingested 80 milligrams of garlic extract a day for twelve weeks lost weight and reduced their BMI significantly.

NUT BUTTER + BANANA

■ Pairing healthy sources of protein and complex carbs does more than aid with muscle recovery post workout. It also keeps you fuller longer. Nut butters are rich in unsaturated fats, which can help deflate a spare tire. And unlike saturated fats, which researchers say turn on certain genes that increase the storage of belly fat, polyunsaturated fats activate genes that shrink fat and improve insulin metabolism. Throwing fiber into the mix increases satiety, warding off mindless snacking.

WHITE TEA + LEMON

■ Who needs Spanx when you can sip on a powerful brew? White tea works in three distinct ways to help strip away fat from your body. A study published in the *Journal of Nutrition and Metabolism* showed that white tea can simultaneously boost lipolysis (the breakdown of fat) and block adipogenesis (the formation of fat cells). Another group of researchers found that the tea is also a rich source of antioxidants that trigger the release of fat from the cells and help speed the liver's ability to turn fat into energy. The vitamin C in just half a lemon can boost fat burning by as much as 25 percent and whittle your waist, according to one study. If there's such a thing as a muffin-top-melting tea, this is it.

RASPBERRIES + WALNUTS

■ In a Canadian study, researchers discovered that those whose diets were supplemented with insoluble fiber had higher levels of ghrelin, a hormone that controls hunger. And a cup of these little ruby jewels has 8 grams of fiber! Insoluble fiber helps feed the healthy bacteria in your gut, triggering production of a fatty acid that reduces inflammation throughout your body. Pairing these fat-burning bullets with good polyunsaturated fats, like those found in walnuts, activate genes that reduce fat storage and improve insulin metabolism. At about 13 grams per 1-ounce serving, walnuts are one of the best dietary sources of those fats.

PEPITAS + GREENS

■ Pepita is the Spanish term for pumpkin seed, and if you consider them just jack-o'-lantern innards, you're in for a treat. One ounce of seeds has 8 grams of protein—more than an egg or almonds—and is rich in flat-belly nutrients like fiber, zinc, and potassium, which are key to muscle building and recovery. Sprinkle them in salads for an extra flat-belly fiber punch.

SWEET POTATOES + GREEK YOGURT

■ When it comes to weight loss, fat burning, and fitness fuel, few foods are more powerful than yogurt. Why opt for Greek over regular? For one, Greek yogurt provides up to double the protein of regular yogurt for the same amount of calories, making it more satiating. Sweet potatoes, on the other hand, are king of slow-digesting carbs, keeping you feeling fuller and energized longer. Among the magic ingredients here are carotenoids, antioxidants that stabilize blood-sugar levels and lower insulin resistance, which prevents calories from being converted into fat. Use a dollop of Greek yogurt in place of sour cream for the combo's fat-frying effects.

WATER + CITRUS FRUITS

■ You see it sitting there every time you're sitting around waiting for a massage. Spa water—a pitcher of ice water with sliced whole lemons, oranges, or grapefruit—is a great substitute for sugary beverages. The citrus peels add d-limonene, a powerful antioxidant that stimulates liver enzymes, helping to rid the body of toxins and flush fat from your system. And don't forget: Delicious smoothies really can help you lose weight!

DARK CHOCOLATE + APPLES

■ Dark chocolate is more than a blissful dessert—it's heavenly for your waistline. A recent study found that the antioxidants in cocoa prevented laboratory mice from gaining excess weight and actually lowered their blood-sugar levels. A separate study at Louisiana State University found that gut microbes in our stomach ferment chocolate into heart-healthy, anti-inflammatory compounds that shut down genes linked to insulin resistance and inflammation. To enhance the effects, try pairing your chocolate (at least 70% cacao) with some apple slices. The fruit speeds up your gut's fermentation process, leading to an even greater reduction in inflammation and weight.

PART-SKIM RICOTTA + BERRIES

■ According to researchers at the University of Tennessee, consuming calcium-rich foods like ricotta can help your body metabolize fat more efficiently. Top it with berries, which contain polyphenols, powerful natural chemicals that can help you lose weight—and even stop fat from forming. In fact, in a recent Texas Woman's University study, researchers found that feeding mice three daily servings of berries decreased the formation of fat cells by up to 73 percent! Mash 1 cup of berries and let them marinate in their own juices for an hour, then spoon them on top of ricotta for a belly-slimming dessert.

CHICKPEAS + OLIVE OIL

■ You might not think of these little beige bullets as a superfood, but it's time to start. High in nutrients and soluble fiber, chickpeas are a prime weight-loss weapon, increasing feelings of satiety by releasing an appetite-suppressing hormone called cholecystokinin. And they blend flawlessly with extra-virgin olive oil (hello hummus!), which may increase blood levels of serotonin, a hormone associated with satiety.

CUCUMBER + APPLE CIDER VINEGAR

■ Cucumbers are about 95 percent water. Not only will they hydrate you, but they also boost your weight-loss efforts thanks to their H_2O content and low calorie count. One medium-size cuke contains only about 45 calories, so you can chomp away guilt-free, but alone they can be kind of a bore. For added flavor and fat-frying, try drizzling them with apple cider vinegar, which has been shown to "switch on" genes that release proteins that break down fat. In a study of 175 overweight Japanese men and women, researchers found that participants who drank 1 or 2 tablespoons of apple cider vinegar daily for twelve weeks significantly lowered their body weight, BMI, visceral fat, and waist circumference.

HOT SAUCE + EGGS

■ Hot sauce is rich in capsaicin, a compound that's proven to suppress appetite and boost thermogenesis—the body's ability to burn fat as energy. A well-cited study by Canadian researchers found that when men ate appetizers with hot sauce (which has zero calories per teaspoon), they ate about 200 fewer calories at later meals than those who did not. Drizzle this fiery condiment over eggs, and fat will sizzle. Eggs are great sources of the weight-loss weapon arginine. Researchers found that administering the amino acid to obese women over twelve weeks resulted in a 7-cm average reduction in waist size and a 6.5-pound average weight loss, according to a recent study published in the *Journal of Dietary Supplements*.

GREEN TEA + MINT

■ In a recent twelve-week study, participants who drank four to five cups of green tea daily, then did a 25-minute workout, lost an average of two more pounds and more belly fat than exercisers who didn't drink tea. What's its magic? The brew contains catechins, a type of antioxidant that triggers the release of fat from fat cells and helps speed the liver's capacity for turning fat into energy. Are you a nighttime eater? Sip a cup of green tea after dinner. The refreshing flavor sends signals to your brain that quash cravings, then tweaks your taste buds so desserts aren't quite so tasty. One study published in *The Journal of Neurological and Orthopaedic Medicine* found that people who sniffed peppermint every two hours lost an average of 5 pounds a month!

BLACK BEAN CHIPS + GUACAMOLE

■ Yes, you read that right; you have our permission to eat chips—so long as they are the nutrient-packed variety. We like Beanitos Black Bean Chips because they pack in more protein and fiber than a "regular" crisp. To boost the staying power of your snack, pair the sea salt–sprinkled treats with a 100-calorie pack of guac. Avocado—the primary ingredient in guacamole—packs healthy monounsaturated fats that contain oleic acid, which helps quiet feelings of hunger.

SPROUTED RAISIN BREAD + PEANUT BUTTER

■ Though this creamy and sweet combination tastes indulgent, nutritionally it's anything but. The raisins in Ezekiel bread provide natural sweetness, which helps nip sugar cravings in the bud, while the vitamin B_6– and manganese-rich whole grains help boost your mood, making it ideal for afternoon slump snack attacks. The nut butter contributes hunger-busting healthy fats and a solid hit of waist-whittling meat-free protein. To keep excess pounds at bay, be sure to buy varieties free of health-harming hydrogenated oils and added sugar.

WHOLE WHEAT CRACKERS + TUNA IN WATER

■ Unlike the majority of crackers you'll find in the grocery store, Triscuit's Baked Whole Grain variety is made with just three ingredients, of which fiber-rich whole-grain wheat is the most abundant. Low-cost, protein-rich tuna makes for a tasty cracker addition and is a solid source of DHA. This type of omega-3 fatty acid down-regulates fat genes in the stomach, preventing fat cells from growing larger and keeping you on track toward your trim-down goal.

BABY CARROTS + HUMMUS

■ In addition to providing healthy fat, fiber, and weight-loss-fueling protein to your plate, this savory duo is packed with belly-filling water, vitamin A (which helps the body synthesize protein), and magnesium, a mineral that helps boost lipolysis, a process by which your body releases fat from its stores. If you tend to snack away from home, look for single-serving hummus containers, and throw your veggies into a plastic snack bag to reap the benefits on the go.

APPLES + PEANUT BUTTER

■ Crunchy, filling (thanks to their high water and fiber content), and packed with nutrients, apples are one of the best weight-loss fruits around. Smearing on all-natural peanut butter adds a creamy texture and slow-digesting, heart-healthy monounsaturated fats to the equation, which keeps your belly satiated until your next meal. Bonus: Peanuts are a top source of genistein and resveratrol, two nutrients that help diminish the action of fat-storage genes.

Chapter 10

THE *SUPER METABOLISM* MOVEMENT PLAN

How to Exercise (or Just Walk!) to Keep Your Metabolism Humming Throughout the Day—Every Day!

FOR A MOMENT I'd like you to imagine a spider. For the record: not the fluorescent red-and-blue, artificially enhanced arachnid that bit Peter Parker's hands and endowed him with the gifts of web-slinging super powers in the Spider-Man films. No, just your average, everyday, eight-legged predator that you'll find occasionally crawling about the garden in your backyard. These are the spiders that spin the beautifully ornate webs that you see portrayed in gauze above household doorways on Halloween. These spiders are largely harmless but no doubt freak out your grandmother—if not you.

When many types of spiders hunt for prey, they opt for a "sit-and-wait" strategy in which they spin their webs and then they let their food come to them. While waiting, they sit there motionless, sometimes for very long periods of time. Yes, it's creepy, but they do it for several reasons. For one, spinning a giant web takes an enormous amount of energy, so they need to conserve what energy they have left. The second is that pouncing on a predator takes a ton of energy, too. And these arachnids, since they need to conserve what energy exists in their little bodies, have abnormally slow resting metabolic rates to keep them alive. That state of motionlessness, when they're not burning up energy and their bodies essentially shut down, is what scientists have termed the super relaxed state (SRX).

And get this: There's increasing evidence that we may do it, too.

In a study published in 2016 in the journal *PLOS One,* researchers led by Roger Cooke, PhD, of the University of California, San Francisco, looked closely at the behavior of myosin, a motor protein in cells that is crucial to muscle function and metabolism in frogs and other animals, including humans. The researchers discovered that in different species—such as spiders—myosin essentially shuts off when the muscles are inactive during the super relaxed state. In other words: When your muscles aren't moving at all—for even short periods—your metabolism is likely taking a breather.

"The large amount of myosin in animals and humans leads to the conclusion," the authors write, "that the equilibrium between the SRX and the DRX [or disordered relaxed state, when mysosin filaments act differently and cells are burning energy] will play a role in whole body metabolism."

Now, this doesn't necessarily mean the solution to a fully

optimized metabolism is living your life on a hamster wheel in constant forward movement. But this groundbreaking research has shined a light on something wildly overlooked in today's day and age: the simple importance of just moving around.

Not hitting up Flywheel for a 45-minute spin class. Not running a marathon. And definitely not training to be a Navy SEAL.

No, I'm talking about simply swinging your arms while you lie on the couch. "Moving throughout the day [is important]," says Stanford's Clyde Wilson, PhD. "Because a simple twitch from your nervous system to muscle is what gets you out of the super relaxed state."

The most cutting edge science on the subject says that stretching, using your jaw muscles to chew gum, fidgeting, standing up when you're sitting down, and even using your muscles *again* to sit down after you've been standing still for a while—will indeed help keep your body burning energy. (That's right: *sitting down* actually boosts your metabolism!)

That leads me to the three tiers of the Movement Plan.

TIER ONE
MOVE MORE THAN A SPIDER

Yes, consider this the bare minimum essential movement requirement for a Super Metabolism. And if it's all you do, you'll still be taking steps for improvement.

According to fitness buff Tim Blake, owner and founder of superfitdads.com, the single biggest thing you can do to get your metabolism firing is to increase your basic movement, or your Non-Exercise Activity Thermogenesis (NEAT). "Basically, that means adding movement to everything you do, whenever and wherever possible," he explains.

This includes simple things like adding fidgeting hands and feet to five hours of desk work. "That racks up an additional caloric expenditure equivalent to running 1.5 miles! Fundamentally, this should be your mantra: Never walk when you can run, never stand when you can walk, never sit when you can stand, never lie down when you can sit."

Simply taking the stairs is the great metabolism-booster, suggests Shari Portnoy of foodlabelnutrition.com. "Even when you're on the escalator, move! People ask why I am skinny and it's because I don't sit still. Anytime you can, just move, take the stairs, walk somewhere, and avoid elevators unless you're carrying a lot."

If you're *really* feeling ambitious about it and are alone, do some squats while you're on that elevator!

Here are a few examples of things you will do every day:

- Stand for five minutes every hour.
- Stand up and sit down in quick succession.
- Walk at least three miles per day. (Varying your speed.)
- Stretch and fidget when possible.
- Clench your abs at your desk for twenty seconds at a time and release.
- Do jumping jacks.
- Take the stairs at work instead of the escalator or elevator.

TIER TWO
GROW YOUR FACTORY

You may recall that I said your body is like a factory that produces a product called energy. Let's say you're determined to burn more energy and therefore burn more fat. There are several ways you can try to accomplish this. You can try to push your current employees to work harder. Unless you're the world's greatest motivator—and capable of inspiring your troops like a general in a Roman epic—this is really hard to do. In terms of your body, it's basically impossible. It probably means cutting your calories so your body works overtime to burn your energy stores. As I've explained, this doesn't work in the long term. No, it actually works against you.

If you're a factory and you want greater output, there's really only one thing you can possibly do: Grow the factory in size. You need to scale, and that means recruiting and hiring more employees to your ranks. And while you can't grow the size of your brain, your liver, your heart, and your other outsize energy burners, you *can* grow your muscles, which burn a lot more energy than your fat does.

"Let me give you another example [with the car metaphor]," says Wilson. "If you're an engine and you've had years of stress and low sleep and you're sedentary, your engine [has shriveled to the] size of a lawn mower engine." And if you're following Tier One—you know, moving around and fidgeting and standing and walking and chewing gum—you're going to improve the efficiency of that lawn mower engine.

But at the end of the day you'll still have a lawn mower engine. If you want to become a Ferrari, you need bigger muscles.

"Then you can double and triple the engine size," he says.

Only then you'll no longer be cutting grass on a John Deere but drag racing down the street in a muscle car like a tattooed badass in the Fast and the Furious films.

Now, this doesn't mean maxing out at the gym. It just means giving your muscles enough resistance so that they can grow and recruit more muscle—which is also largely thanks to the protein you'll be ingesting in the Super Metabolism Diet. Here is a sampling of some of the exercise moves you'll find in the Super Metabolism Movement Plan:

Do-Anywhere Body-Weight Moves:
- Push-ups
- Squats
- Lunges
- Crunches
- Planks
- Wall Sits

At-the-Gym Weight Moves:

- Bench Press (with Dumbbells or Bar)
- Dead Lift
- Pull-ups and Dips
- Power Cleans
- Rows
- Kettlebell Swings

TIER THREE
MAKE YOUR BODY MORE EFFICIENT

When you've built your factory in size and you've improved your muscle-to-fat ratio, you'll find that you're burning more calories than you ever have before. But you can *still* do better to improve your factory and boost your metabolism. Now, that doesn't mean necessarily getting even *bigger* and looking like a person on the cover of a muscle magazine or the Incredible Hulk. It means making your body more efficient, and the best way of achieving peak efficiency is to add intensity to your routine.

You've probably heard of the term "high-intensity interval training" (HIIT) before. At its most basic, it means doing short bursts of really intense exercise—like throwing ropes at the gym, doing all-out sprints (on foot or on a bike), performing Burpees or mountain climbers, trying the VersaClimber at your gym, or anything else that is really, really hard and you can only perform for a relatively short amount of time—and then resting for a brief period of time (like, say, five or ten seconds), and then going at it again. "This places a high metabolic demand on the body, burns lots of calories in a short amount of time, produces a high post-workout calorie burn, and helps to improve one's fitness level," explains Kathleen Trotter, personal trainer and author of *Finding Your Fit.* "Plus, intervals are a fantastic workout regardless of your fitness level; you adapt the interval intensity to fit your current capacity."

Don't get me wrong: HIIT is hard. But studies are showing that it's probably the single most effective form of exercise you can be doing—and if you've built up your muscle mass, HIIT will unlock the full forces of your metabolism.

A study conducted by the Mayo Clinic and published in the journal *Cell Metabolism* in 2017 found that HIIT exercise can actually *slow down* your body's aging process on a cellular level. As I've described in this book, your muscles are the home to so many of your energy-burning mitochondria. As you age and your metabolism slows down, your mitochondria slow down as well. But the researchers discovered evidence that right after super intense workout, mitochondria came back to life—in the HIIT group of participants in the study, mitochondrial function improved by 69 percent among older people, and by 49 percent among younger people.

The study bolsters what a lot of experts already know: that rapid-fire workouts supercharge your body in countless ways. Unlike doing "steady-state" cardio, in which you head out for a leisurely jog or casually climb a Stairmaster, high-intensity workouts ignite your body's stress response. Everything from your blood pressure to your heart rate spikes. Your immune system and central nervous system kick into high gear. You start inhaling more and more oxygen to spread to your cells. Blood starts flowing to your muscles and your body instantly starts burning up all of that glucose in your blood—meaning you'll stave off weight gain and bring your endocrine system back into the balance. Physically speaking, it's the closest thing you can do to running into a phone booth and emerging afterward with a cape and giant "S" on your chest.

"If people are looking to improve performance in the most time-effective way, and if they're looking to improve health in the most time effective way, then I think incorporating interval training is a very good strategy," says Martin Gibala, PhD, a professor of kinesiology at Canada's McMaster University—and widely regarded as one of the world's foremost experts on high-intensity exercise. Over the years Gibala has performed several landmark studies on their efficacy and has done more than any single person to raise awareness of short, intense workouts.

"The idea of boosting intensity—which can result in greater improvements in cardiorespiratory fitness—is important not only if you're an athlete but also if you're an average, everyday [person] looking to maintain a higher quality of life," he says. "For a higher health span, not just life span. We need to worry about health span, and that's basically optimal physical activity in order to maintain your health."

Dr. Gibala isn't the only high-profile evangelist of HIIT. In Norway, a scientist named Ulrik Wisløff, PhD, introduced the breakthrough concept of your "fitness age" in a landmark 2013 study. Having studied the biomarkers of more than forty-six hundred men and women, he developed a proprietary way of calculating *physically* how old you are—as opposed to simply "how old you are" in terms of age.

Let me explain.

According to Wisløff, if you're forty years old, he can determine through a few tests and biomarkers if you actually have the body of an average forty-year-old—or if your body is, in reality, better or worse off than the average body for someone your same age. In other words, yes: You *can* be sixty years old and have the "fitness age" of a thirty-year-old—if you're in good enough shape, and vice versa. Explaining his formula is quite complicated—it all comes down to your body's cardiorespiratory fitness, or its ability to use oxygen—but here's the major, earth-shattering point: Wisløff found that the surest way to stave off the grim effects of aging is to engage in high-intensity workouts.

If that sounds like something you're interested in, here are some examples of moves you could be doing:

- Burpees
- Box Jumps
- Broad Jump
- Jump Squats
- Power Squats
- Squat Thrusts
- Mountain Climbers
- Sprints
- Snap Kicks
- Side-to-side Hops

Chapter 11

THE *SUPER METABOLISM* WORKOUTS

Easy to Hard, Full-Body Exercises That Will Get Your Metabolism Running Hotter Than Ever!

I'VE DEVISED three tiers in the Super Metabolism Movement Plan, and they're arranged in ascending order of difficulty. If you only feel like Tier One—moving, walking, standing—that's great! Combined with the Super Metabolism Diet you're still guaranteed to lose weight, feel better, and boost your metabolism. If you opt for Tier Two—strength training—you'll be building more muscle, which means your metabolism will be getting an extra rocket booster of help. If you opt for Tier Three, you'll be burning fat, feeling better, and living longer than you ever imagined.

One caveat: Don't skip from one to three if you're not conditioned for it. "In the long run, it's better to get into shape and be genuinely prepared [for high-intensity activity]," says Robert S. Herbst, personal trainer, coach, and powerlifter. "For example, first your body may not be ready for a big workout first thing in the morning since its core temperature is low and muscles and tendons are stiff. It's better to do some stretching—and perhaps even eat a breakfast of protein and carbohydrates—so that the metabolism is on an even footing."

At the end of the day, you're like a spider. If you're doing nothing, you're burning nothing. And that's the most dangerous workout of them all.

TIER ONE WORKOUTS

If you are overweight and don't work out regularly, here are all of the greatest workouts to get you started on the path to a leaner body and a healthier lifestyle.

THE JUMP-START YOUR METABOLISM MORNING WORKOUT

Jumping Jacks: Jump, while reaching your arms out 90 degrees to your sides as your legs spread. When you jump your legs back in, clap your hands together in front of you.
30 seconds

Plank: Get into push-up position and then bend your elbows so your forearms lie flat on the floor. Brace your abs and hold the position.
30 seconds

Sumo Squat: Stand with feet outside shoulder width and turn your toes out 45 degrees. Raise your arms up for balance as you squat down. Push your knees out on the descent and drive your heels into the floor as you come up.
30 seconds

Repeat 3 times.

PLANK

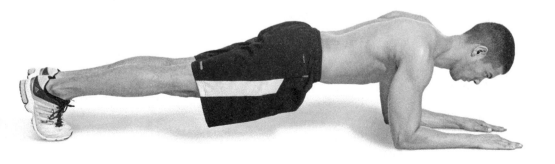

THE 45-MINUTE METABOLISM WALKING WORKOUT

6 minutes—warm-up of easy effort

60 seconds—walk fast

2 minutes—walk slower, at an easy effort

60 seconds—walk fast

2 minutes—walk slower, at an easy effort

60 seconds—walk fast

2 minutes—walk slower, at an easy effort

60 seconds—walk fast

2 minutes—walk slower, at an easy effort

60 seconds—walk fast

2 minutes—walk slower, at an easy effort

60 seconds—walk fast

2 minutes—walk slower, at an easy effort

60 seconds—walk fast

2 minutes—walk slower, at an easy effort

60 seconds—walk fast

2 minutes—walk slower, at an easy effort

60 seconds—walk fast

2 minutes—walk slower, at an easy effort

60 seconds—walk fast

2 minutes—walk slower, at an easy effort

60 seconds—walk fast

2 minutes—walk slower, at an easy effort

60 seconds—walk fast

2 minutes—walk slower, at an easy effort

3 minutes—cooldown

THE MIDDAY METABOLISM STAIRWELL CARDIO WORKOUT

- Perform every exercise for 20 seconds each and rest for anywhere from 1 to 3 minutes between each circuit (until you've got your wind back). Repeat the entire workout 3 times.
- Walk two steps at a time up the stairs. Jog back down.
- Run up the stairs one step at a time. Jog back down.
- Hop on one foot one step (or two steps for more difficulty) at a time. Jog back down.
- Bunny hop with both feet up three steps at a time. Jog back down.
- Rest.

THE 5-MINUTE AT-YOUR-DESK WORKOUT

- This workout will engage in isometrics—or contracting and flexing your muscles for sustained periods of time—at your desk. (Remember: When it comes to your metabolism, every movement counts.) Perform this routine 3 times, resting for 10 seconds in between each exercise:
- Holding a pen, clench your forearms and your fists as hard as you can for a full 20 seconds. Then release.
- Squeeze your glutes (or butt cheeks!) together as hard as you can, ensuring that you rise out of your seat for at least an inch. Hold for 20 seconds and then release.
- Squeeze your entire body below the neck for a full 20 seconds and then release.
- Relax for 30 seconds.

TIER TWO WORKOUTS

If you're ready to build muscle and take your fitness to the next level, here are the simplest and most effective strength training exercises to get you started immediately.

THE DO-ANYWHERE BODY-WEIGHT WORKOUT

DIRECTIONS

Set a timer for 10 minutes and complete as many circuits as you can at an easy pace.

1) PRISONER SQUAT

Place your hands behind your head, interlacing your fingers. Stand with your feet shoulder width and your toes turned slightly out. Squat as low as you can.

2) SEAL JUMP

Perform a jumping jack, reaching your arms out 90 degrees to your sides as your legs spread. When you jump your legs back in, clap your hands together in front of you.

3) PUSH-UP

Place your hands on the floor at shoulder width. Keeping your abs braced and your body in a straight line, squeeze your shoulder blades together and lower your body until your chest is an inch above the floor.

4) LATERAL JUMP

Jump to your right side and land on your right foot. Rebound off your right foot and jump back to your left to begin the next rep.

PRISONER SQUAT

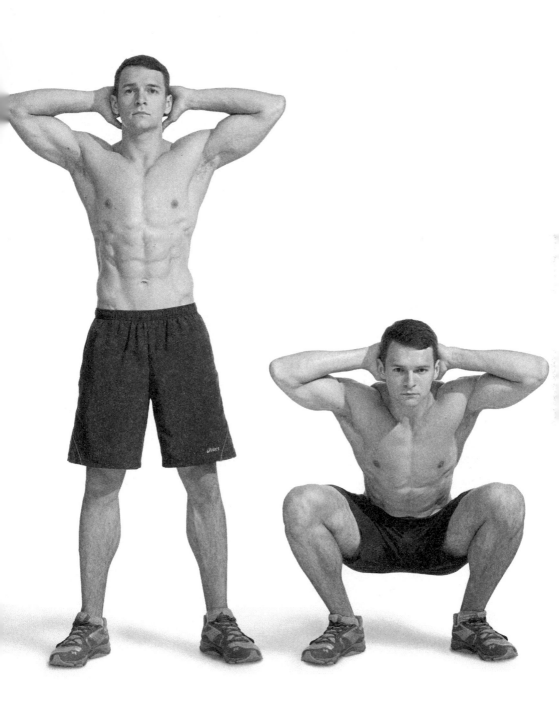

THE FULL-BODY WEIGHT ROOM WORKOUT

Complete all five sets for the squat and then perform the overhead press and weighted pull-up in alternating fashion. That is, complete a set of the press, rest, then do a set of the pull-up, rest again, and repeat until you've finished all five sets for each.

1) SQUAT

SETS: 5 **REPS:** 5 **REST:** 120 sec.

■ Set up in a squat rack or cage. Grasp the bar as far apart as is comfortable and step under it. Squeeze your shoulder blades together and nudge the bar out of the rack. Step back and stand with your feet shoulder-width apart and your toes turned slightly outward. Take a deep breath and bend your hips back and then bend your knees to lower your body as far as you can without losing the arch in your lower back. Push your knees outward as you descend. Extend your hips to come back up, continuing to push your knees outward.

2A) OVERHEAD PRESS

SETS: 5 **REPS:** 5 **REST:** 60 sec.

■ Set the bar up in a squat rack or cage and grasp it just outside shoulder width. Take the bar off the rack and hold it at shoulder level with your forearms perpendicular to the floor. Squeeze the bar and brace your abs. Press the bar overhead, pushing your head forward and shrugging your traps as the bar passes your face.

2B) WEIGHTED PULL-UP

SETS: 5 **REPS:** 5 **REST:** 60 sec.

■ Attach a weighted belt to your waist or hold a dumbbell between your feet. Hang from a pull-up bar with your hands just outside shoulder width. Pull yourself up until your chin is over the bar. If you can't complete your reps with weight, it's okay to use body weight alone.

THE FULL-BODY FAT-LOSS MUSCLE BUILDER

Perform the first exercise (Swiss-Ball Plank) as straight sets—do one set, rest, then the other, rest. Exercises 2A through 2D are done as a complex, so choose one pair of dumbbells and use it for each move. It should be a load that allows you more than the required reps on your weakest exercise in the series. Perform six reps for each of the exercises in succession. Rest 90 seconds and repeat until all sets are completed.

For exercises 3A through 3D, adjust your equipment and loads as necessary but perform them in the same circuit fashion. If you choose to repeat the workout, vary the sets and reps you perform on these last four exercises each session. This will help you to continue milking gains from the circuit for months on end. Rotate between 3 sets of 10 reps, 4 sets of 5 reps, and 2 sets of 15 reps.

1) SWISS-BALL PLANK
SETS: 2 **REPS:** "Stir" for 30–45 seconds **REST:** 60–90 sec.

■ Place a Swiss ball on the floor and get into push-up position with your hands on it. Now lower your forearms to rest on the ball, keeping your entire body in a straight line with abs braced. Use your elbows to roll the ball in a circular motion, clockwise and then counterclockwise, as if you were stirring a pot.

2A) DUMBBELL ROMANIAN DEAD LIFT
SETS: 3–5 **REPS:** 6 **REST:** 0 sec.

■ Hold a dumbbell in each hand and stand with feet hip-width apart. Push your hips back and, keeping your lower back in its natural arch, bend your torso forward. Lower your body until you feel a stretch in your hamstrings, bending slightly at the knees as needed. Squeeze your glutes as you come back up.

2B) ALTERNATING DUMBBELL ROW
SETS: 3–5 **REPS:** 6 (each side) **REST:** 0 sec.

■ Bend forward at the hips as you did in the Romanian dead lift and row one dumbbell to your side. Lower it and repeat on the other side.

2C) DUMBBELL HIGH PULL
SETS: 3–5 **REPS:** 6 **REST:** 0 sec.
■ Hold dumbbells in front of your thighs and bend your knees and hips so the weights hang just above your knees. Explosively extend your hips as if jumping and pull the weights up to shoulder level with your elbows wide apart, as in an upright row.

2D) FRONT SQUAT TO PRESS
SETS: 3–5 **REPS:** 6 **REST:** 90 sec.
■ Hold the dumbbells at shoulder level and stand with your feet shoulder-width apart. Squat as low as you can without losing the arch in your lower back. Come back up and press the weights overhead.

3A) SNATCH-GRIP RACK DEAD LIFT
SETS: 3 **REPS:** 10 **REST:** 0 sec.
■ Set up as you would to deadlift, only do so in a power rack, resting the bar on the safety rods at about two inches below your knees. Grasp the bar wide, hands about double shoulder-width apart. Extend your hips and stand up, pulling the bar to in front of your thighs.

3B) ALTERNATING DUMBBELL BENCH PRESS
SETS: 3 **REPS:** 10 (each side) **REST:** 0 sec.
■ Lie back on a flat bench holding dumbbells. Press them both over your chest and then lower one of them to your side. Press it up and then lower the other hand. That's one rep.

3C) DUMBBELL LUNGE
SETS: 3 **REPS:** 10 (each side) **REST:** 0 sec.
■ Stand with your feet hip-width apart, holding a dumbbell in each hand. Step forward with one leg and lower your body until your rear knee nearly touches the floor and your front thigh is parallel to the floor.

3D) INVERTED ROW
SETS: 3 **REPS:** 10 **REST:** 90 sec.
■ Set a barbell in a power rack (or use a Smith machine) at about hip height. Lie underneath it and grab it with hands about shoulder-width apart. Hang from the bar so your body forms a straight line. Squeeze your shoulder blades together and pull yourself up until your back is fully contracted.

ALTERNATING DUMBBELL BENCH PRESS

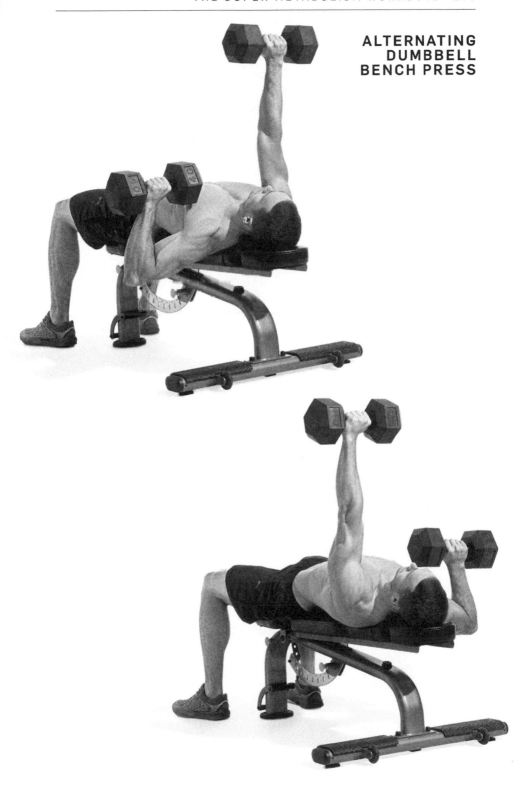

THE SUPER BODY-WEIGHT WORKOUT

DIRECTIONS

Perform the exercises as a circuit, completing a set of each in turn and resting as little as possible between sets. Repeat for 10 circuits (until you're doing only 1 rep per exercise).

1) JUMP SQUAT

REPS: 10 to 1 **REST:** 0 sec.

■ Stand with feet shoulder width apart and squat down until your thighs are about parallel to the floor but no deeper. Jump as high as you can. Land with soft knees and begin the next rep. Perform 10 reps. Each time you repeat the circuit, perform one less rep. So the next round you'll do 9 reps, then 8, and so on down to 1 rep.

2) PULL-UP

REPS: 10 to 1 **REST:** 0 sec.

■ Hang from a pull-up bar, jungle gym, or tree limb and pull yourself up until your chin is higher than your hands. Perform 10 reps down to 1 as described above.

3) DIP

REPS: 10 to 1 **REST:** 0 sec.

■ Suspend yourself over parallel bars and then lower your body until your upper arms are parallel to the floor. Perform 10 reps down to 1.

THE ONE-DUMBBELL (OR KETTLEBELL) WORKOUT

DIRECTIONS

The workout consists of two circuits. In Circuit 1, you'll perform the exercises in sequence for 6 reps each. Complete as many rounds as possible in 6 minutes, and then rest 1 minute. Repeat twice more and then rest 2 minutes.

Go on to Circuit 2, and perform as directed below.

CIRCUIT 1

1) ONE-ARM SNATCH

REPS: 6 (each side) **REST:** 0 sec.

■ Hold a kettlebell in front of your thighs with your right hand and stand with feet between hip- and shoulder-width apart. Keep your torso as upright as possible and bend your knees until the weight hangs at mid-shin level—maintain the arch in your lower back. Jump, extending your hips explosively, and raise the weight straight up your body. When it gets to your chest, flip your wrist and "catch" the bell overhead with arm extended.

2) KETTLEBELL PRESS-OUT

REPS: 6 **REST:** 0 sec.

■ Hold the weight close to your chest at shoulder level with both hands on the handle and palms facing each other. Squat down as deeply as you can and then press the bell straight out in front of you with arms extended. Bring it back to your shoulders and repeat for 5 more reps while maintaining the squat position.

3) HARD-STYLE KETTLEBELL SWING

REPS: 6 **REST:** 0 sec.

■ Stand with feet hip-width apart and the weight on the floor. Grasp the kettlebell with both hands (palms facing you) and, keeping your lower back flat, extend your hips to raise it off the floor and between your legs. From there, take a deep breath and bend your hips back, allowing the weight to swing back between your legs. Explosively extend your hips and exhale—allowing the momentum to swing the weight up to your shoulders. Control the descent but use the momentum to begin the next rep.

CIRCUIT 2

TURKISH GETUP

■ Perform 1 rep with the weight in your right hand and then immediately switch hands and repeat. Switch back to your right hand and do 2 reps. Then do 2 on your left. Continue adding a rep in this fashion until you're up to 5 on each side. Without rest, reverse the process and work back down to 1 rep.

Lie on your back on the floor holding a kettlebell with your right hand over your chest. Bend your right knee 90 degrees and plant your foot on the floor. Brace your abs and raise your torso off the floor. Use your left elbow for support. Now use your right foot to raise your hips off the floor. Sweep out your left leg back and rest on your left knee. Come up to a standing position, and then reverse the motion to return to the floor. Note that the foot that rests on the floor changes with the hand that's holding the weight (when you perform the getup with the left hand, your left foot will lie flat).

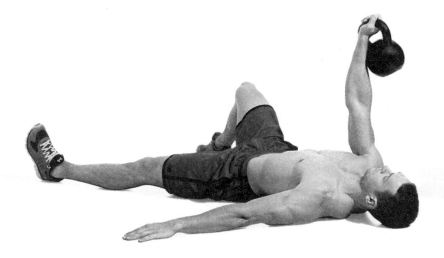

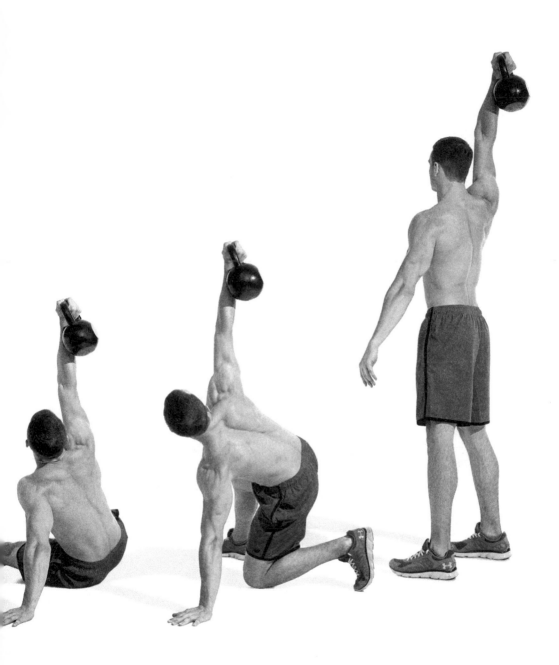

THE ALL-STAR ABS WORKOUT

■ The secret to firming your abs fast (so you can show them off ASAP) is to crank up the intensity. These exercises do it by either adding resistance, challenging your coordination, or both. The result: You'll work harder than you would during an ordinary crunch and hit all your middle muscles, scoring sexy definition stat!

YOU'LL NEED
A 3- to 6-pound medicine ball, a pair of 3- or 5-pound dumbbells, a stability ball, and a resistance band.

ROPE CLIMB
(A mat is optional.)

■ Lie faceup with your knees bent and feet flat on the ground. Bend your arms and tuck your elbows close to your sides, about an inch off the ground; make loose fists with your hands. Raise your head and shoulder blades while reaching your left arm slightly to the right and up, extending your fingers as if you were reaching for a rope to pull it down [shown]. Lower your left arm and reach with your right arm while you rotate slightly to the left to complete 1 rep.

TIP: Imagine the rope is dangling over the center of your chest—that's the direction you should reach.

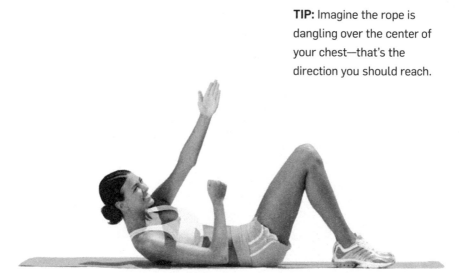

PIKE PRESS-UP

■ Hold a dumbbell with both hands and lie faceup, legs extended at a 45-degree angle off the ground. Extend arms straight up over your chest. Lift your head and shoulder blades, pressing the dumbbell straight up [shown]. Lower to starting position.

TIP: To make this move easier, extend your legs straight up over your hips; lowering your legs closer to the floor will make it more challenging.

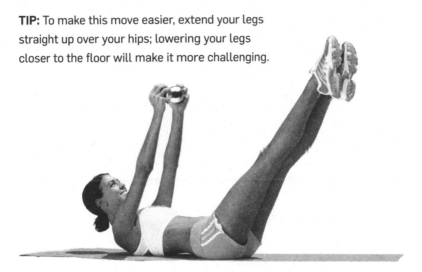

MEDICINE-BALL DOUBLE CRUNCH

■ Lie faceup with your knees bent over your hips and squeeze a medicine ball between your calves and upper thighs. (If you don't have a medicine ball, do the move without weight.) Place your hands behind your head. Simultaneously lift your head, shoulder blades, and hips [shown]. Lower to starting position.

TIP: Think about lifting your butt (not your knees).

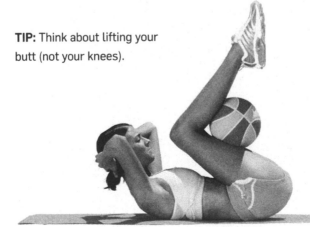

DUMBBELL REACH

■ Hold a dumbbell in your left hand and lie faceup with your knees bent and feet flat on the ground. Place your right hand on your belly and extend your left arm straight up in line with your shoulder. Lift your head and shoulders as you slightly draw your left shoulder toward your right knee [shown]. Lower and repeat. Switch sides to complete the set.

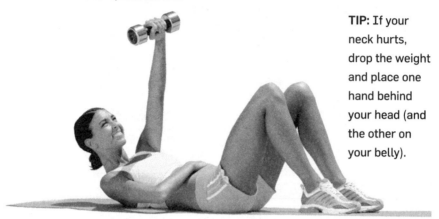

TIP: If your neck hurts, drop the weight and place one hand behind your head (and the other on your belly).

ONE-LEG KNEE-IN

■ Get in plank position with your shins on a stability ball. Raise your left leg a few inches. Press your right foot into the ball as you bend your right knee, rolling the ball toward your hands [shown]. Extend your right leg to return to starting position and repeat. Switch sides to complete the set.

TIP: Don't have a stability ball? Hold plank position and draw one knee toward your chest, alternating knees each rep.

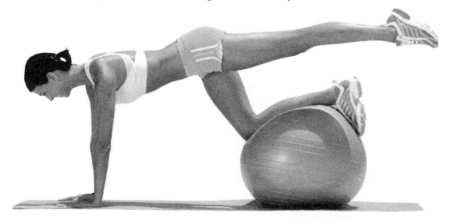

BAND PULL

■ Anchor one end of a resistance band around a sturdy object about a foot off the ground and grasp the other in your right hand. Lie faceup with your left hand on your belly and extend your right arm behind you; adjust your position so the band is taut **A**. Keeping your right arm next to your head, curl your shoulder blades off the ground. **B**. Hold for one count, then slowly lower to start position and repeat. Switch sides to complete set.

TIP: If your neck feels strained, place your free hand behind your head to support it.

A

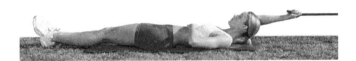

B

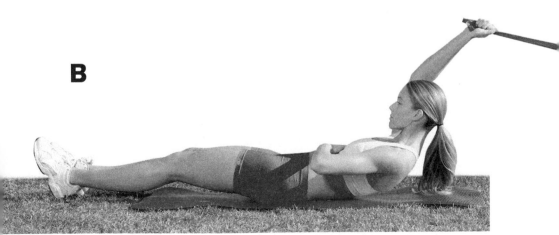

DUMBBELL ROLL-UP

■ Hold a dumbbell in each hand and lie faceup, arms extended over your chest, palms facing forward. Keeping your arms straight up, slowly raise your upper body **A** until your torso is perpendicular to the ground **B**. Roll down to starting position.

A

TIP: Move as slowly as you can, curling one vertebra at a time up and then down.

B

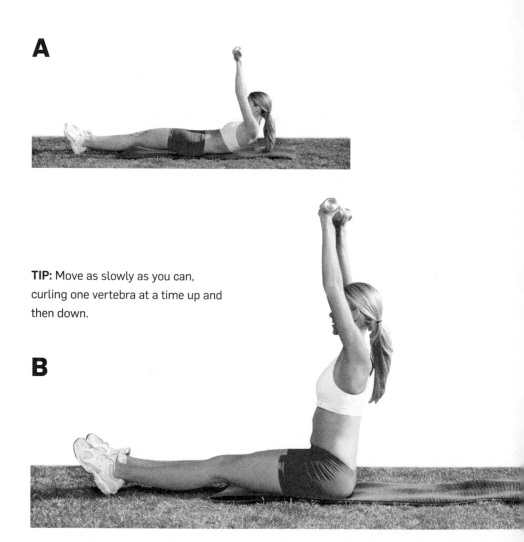

BALL TWIST

■ Hold one end of a dumbbell in both hands and lie with your shoulders centered on a stability ball. Place your feet shoulder-width apart on the ground and extend your arms over your chest so the dumbbell is vertical. Lift your hips so your body is straight from your head to your knees **A**. Keeping your arms straight and hips raised, rotate your torso to the left (ball will move under you) and lower your weight until your arms are parallel to the ground and your left shoulder is centered on the ball **B**. Return to starting position and repeat to the right side to complete 1 rep.

A

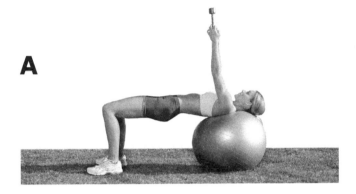

B

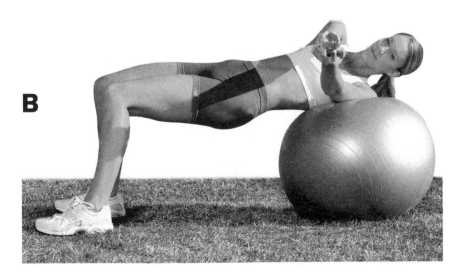

TIER THREE WORKOUTS

If you're ready to improve the efficiency of your muscles, here are the best high-intensity exercises for making you as fighting fit as possible.

THE TOTAL-BODY 20-MINUTE WORKOUT

■ The workout is broken into 6 circuits. It may look long, but the whole routine will take only 20 minutes. Perform the circuits in order, repeating where noted. Your rest between exercises should be only as long as it takes to transition between moves. Repeat this workout up to four times a week on nonconsecutive days.

CIRCUIT A

1) TREADMILL RUN/WALK

■ Walk 1 minute and then sprint 1 minute.

2) DUMBBELL FLY

REPS: 8–10

■ Lie back on a flat bench with a dumbbell in each hand. Keep a slight bend in your elbows and spread your arms wide, lowering the weights until they're even with your chest. Flex your pecs and lift the weights back to the starting position.

3) PUSH-UP

REPS: No more than 15

■ Place your hands on the floor at shoulder width. Keeping your abs braced and your body in a straight line, squeeze your shoulder blades together and lower your body until your chest is an inch above the floor.

4) PLANK

REPS: Hold for 30 seconds

■ Get into push-up position and then lower your forearms to the floor. Brace your abs and hold the position.

Repeat circuit once more.

CIRCUIT B

1) PULL-UP
REPS: As many as possible
■ Hang from a pull-up bar with hands outside shoulder width. Pull yourself up until your chin is over the bar.

2) DUMBBELL LATERAL RAISE
REPS: 12–15
■ Hold a dumbbell in each hand and stand with palms facing your sides. Raise the weights up and out 90 degrees until your arms are parallel to the floor.

3) LYING DUMBBELL SKULL CRUSHER
REPS: 10–12
■ Lie back on a flat bench with a dumbbell in each hand. Hold the weights over your chest, palms facing each other. Bend your elbows and lower the weights to the sides of your head.

4) SIDE-TO-SIDE HOP
REPS: Continue for 30 seconds
■ Place something small on the floor to act as a hurdle and jump over it side to side. Minimize your contact with the floor.
Repeat circuit once more

CIRCUIT C

1) DUMBBELL LUNGE
REPS: 20 (each leg)
■ Stand with your feet hip-width apart, holding a dumbbell in each hand. Step forward with one leg and lower your body until your rear knee nearly touches the floor and your front thigh is parallel to the floor.

2) BURPEE
REPS: 10
■ Stand with feet shoulder-width apart and bend down and place your hands on the floor. Now shoot your legs behind you fast so you end up in the top of a push-up position. Jump your legs back up so they land between your hands and then stand up quickly.
Move on to Circuit D.

CIRCUIT D

1) DUMBBELL PULLOVER

REPS: 10

■ Lie on a bench holding a dumbbell by one end over your face. Lower the weight behind your head so you feel a stretch in your lats. Pull the weight back over your face.

2) HOP ONTO BENCH

REPS: 20

■ Stand behind a bench or low box and hop up onto it. Step down and repeat.
Repeat circuit once more.

CIRCUIT E

1) DUMBBELL CURL

REPS: 15

■ Hold a dumbbell in each hand and, keeping your upper arms in place, curl the weights.

2) LATERAL BAND WALK

REPS: 20

■ Wrap an elastic band around your ankles and step sideways for 20 feet and then come back, keeping tension on your legs throughout.
Repeat circuit once more.

CIRCUIT F

1) STEP-UP

REPS: Repeat for 30 seconds

■ Place one foot on a bench. Step up onto the bench but don't rest the trailing leg on it.

2) LEG LIFT

REPS: To failure

■ Lie on the floor and hold on to a bench or the legs of a heavy chair for support. Keep your legs straight and raise them up until they're vertical. Lower them back down but stop just short of the floor to keep tension on your abs before the next rep.

THE SUPER SPRINTING WORKOUT

DIRECTIONS

Perform 8 to 10 sprints of 20–40 yards. Run at slightly less than your absolute top speed for safety. Rest as needed between sets—keep your heart rate elevated but allow yourself enough recovery that you can go fast. Warm up thoroughly beforehand, and run a few practice sprints at a low intensity (but go a little faster each time).

If you're new to sprinting or haven't done it in a while, do your sprints on a hill. Start with 5 and run only at a moderate pace and build up from there.

Land on the balls of your feet as you sprint—not your heels. Your front foot should land directly beneath you (unless the hill is especially steep). Your arms should pump vigorously forward and backward as you run, and never cross the midline of your body. Let your hands come up to face level and then back to your pockets, but no farther. Keep your shoulders and hips level so there's no side-to-side rotation in your torso.

THE HIIT ROWING MACHINE WORKOUT

DIRECTIONS

Sit on the rower's seat and adjust the foot height for the size of your feet. Strap your feet onto the rower's foot plates—the strap should be at or above the ball of your foot. Set the drag on the machine to between 3 and 5 (this best simulates rowing on water), grasp the handle, and sit back so your torso is almost vertical. You should feel pressure on the balls of your feet and your heels should be raised slightly off the foot plate. This is the "catch" position.

Drive with your legs, dropping your heels to the foot plate, to push your body back and then row the handle to your sternum. Row as fast as possible for all intervals, but take twice as long to return your body back to the catch position after each row stroke. Maintain this rhythm.

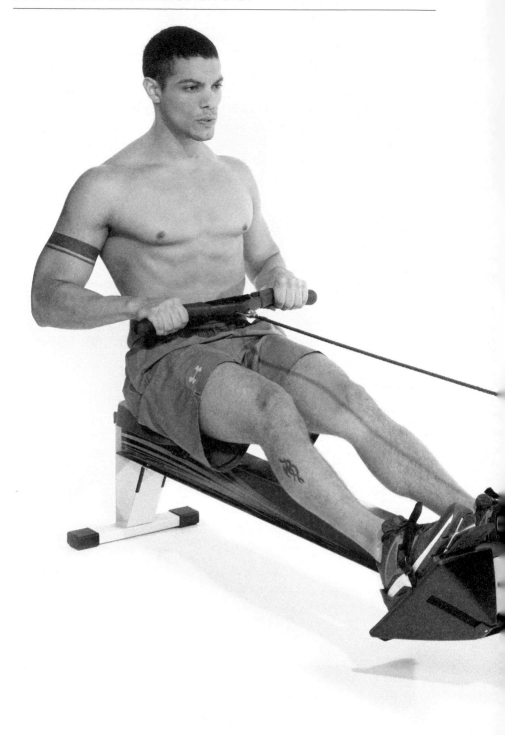

PERFORM THE FOLLOWING INTERVALS:

- **Row 100 meters;** rest 30 seconds
- **Row 200 meters;** rest 30 seconds
- **Row 300 meters;** rest 30 seconds
- **Row 400 meters;** rest 30 seconds
- **Row 500 meters;** rest 30 seconds
- **Row 400 meters;** rest 30 seconds
- **Row 300 meters;** rest 30 seconds
- **Row 200 meters;** rest 30 seconds
- **Row 100 meters;** rest 30 seconds

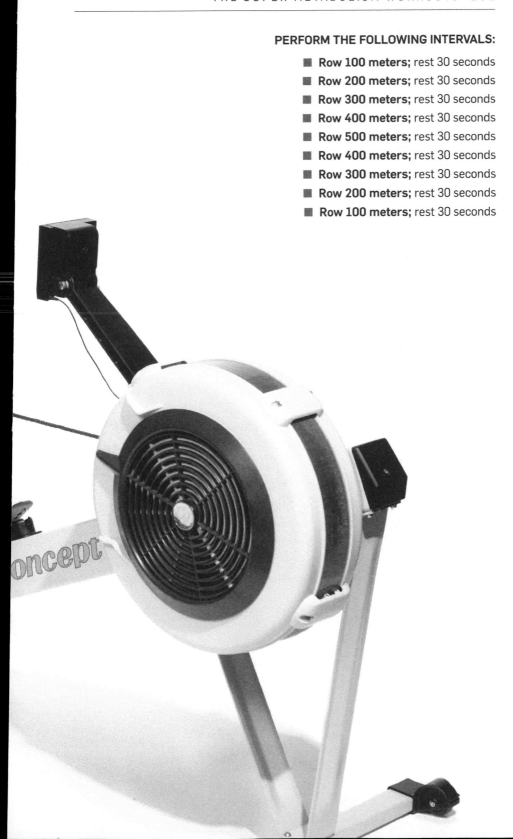

THE SUPER TREADMILL HIIT WORKOUT

The workout breaks down into blocks of brisk walking, jogging, and light walking for active recovery. You'll begin your runs somewhat fatigued from the steep incline walking you do beforehand, and this will take your heart rate near its max. Before you burn out, you back off to a lighter pace to catch your breath, and then the cycle begins again.

DIRECTIONS

BLOCK 1
■ Set the treadmill on a 9-degree incline and walk 60 seconds.
■ Decrease the incline to 3 degrees and run at the fastest speed you can maintain for 120 seconds.
■ Slow down to a walk for 60 seconds.

BLOCK 2
■ Increase the incline to 8 degrees and walk for 60 seconds.
■ Decrease the incline to 4 degrees and run at the fastest speed you can maintain for 120 seconds.
■ Reduce the incline to 3 degrees and walk 60 seconds.

BLOCK 3
■ Raise the incline to 7 degrees and walk 60 seconds.
■ Lower the incline to 5 degrees and run as fast as you can maintain for 120 seconds.
■ Reduce the incline to 3 degrees and walk 60 seconds.

BLOCK 4
■ Increase the incline to 4 degrees and run 4 minutes.
■ Walk on the 4-degree incline for 5 minutes.

THE SUPER 4-MINUTE WORKOUT

DIRECTIONS

Perform burpees for 20 seconds. Don't worry about counting reps—just set a timer and get as many in as you can. Afterward, rest 10 seconds, and then repeat for 4 minutes. Over time, you can progress the length of the work interval, but keep the ratio of work to rest at two to one (so if you build up to doing burpees for 30 seconds, rest 15 seconds between sets).

You can also increase the length of the workout. But we wouldn't do that if we were you. You'll see.

BURPEE

■ Stand with feet shoulder-width apart and bend down and place your hands on the floor. Now shoot your legs behind you fast so you end up in the top of a push-up position. Jump your legs back up so they land between your hands and then jump up quickly.

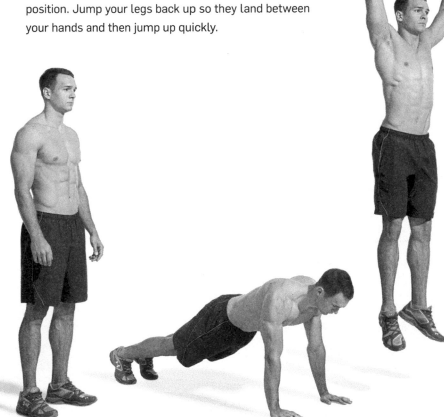

THE ZERO BELLY HIIT BODY-WEIGHT WORKOUT

■ As I first reported in my book *Zero Belly Diet*, this amazing high-intensity workout involves nothing more than body-weight exercises, thus maximizing aerobic efficiency while working your musculature. It's surprisingly intense—so intense that four sessions of just 4 minutes of it per week will do the trick!

EVERY EXERCISE IS TO BE PERFORMED AS FAST AS POSSIBLE WITHOUT LOSING FORM.

3 minutes—Warm up on a stationary cardio machine, do jumping jacks, or jog in place.

20 seconds—Run in Place (high knees)

10 seconds—Rest

20 seconds—Mountain Climbers

10 seconds—Rest

20 seconds—Skater Jumps (side-to-side, mimicking a skater's stride)

10 seconds—Rest

20 seconds—Push-ups (elbows close to sides of body)

10 seconds—Rest

Repeat work/rest cycle once.

3 minutes—Cool down with any of above warm-up movements for 5 minutes.

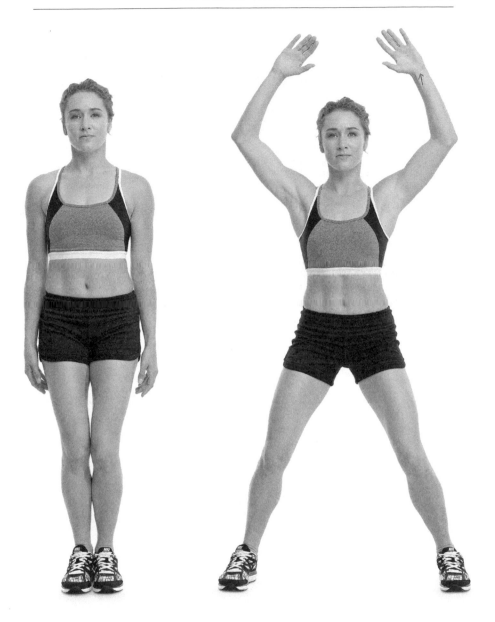

1. WARM-UP JUMPING JACKS

■ Stand with your feet slightly less than shoulder-width apart, hands at your sides. Jump into the air, spreading your feet as wide as you can while swinging your arms out to the sides and bringing your hands together over your head. Immediately jump back up and return your hands and feet to the starting position. That's one Jumping Jack. Repeat at a comfortable pace without stopping for the duration of your warm-up.

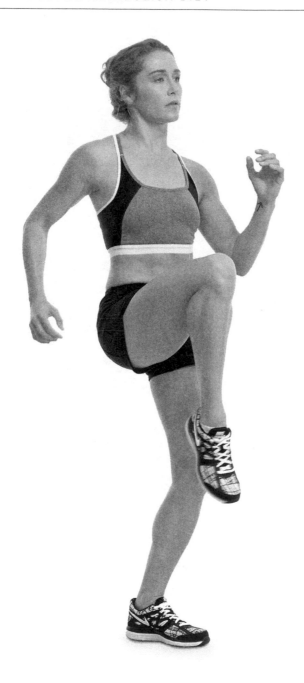

2. RUN IN PLACE (HIGH KNEES)

■ Run in place, bringing your knees up as high as you can and pumping your legs as quickly as you can, for 20 seconds.

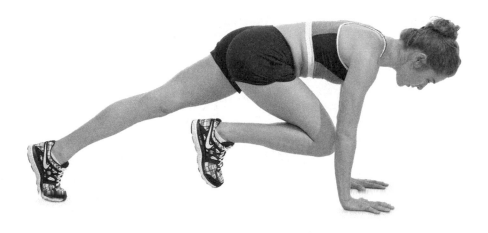

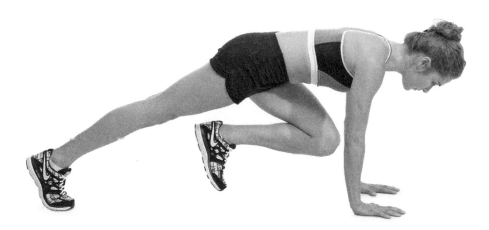

3. MONTAIN CLIMBERS

■ Get into a push-up position, with your arms straight. Raise your hips as you bring one knee up toward your chest, then bring it back to the start position as you bring the other knee forward. The movement should be dynamic: Rather than simply moving one leg followed by the other, get a rhythm going akin to jogging, where both feet are off the floor for a brief moment.

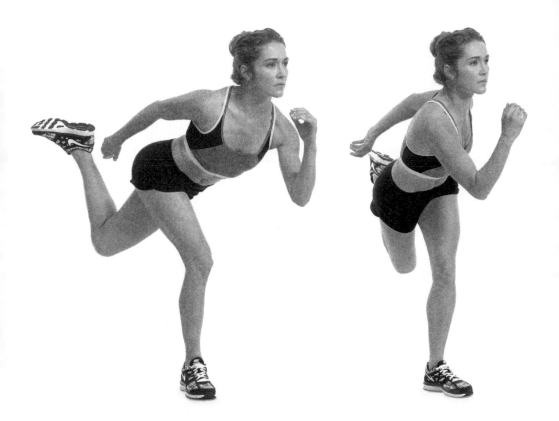

4. SKATER JUMPS

■ From a crouched position with your feet close together, take a sideways leap to your left, landing on your left foot, with your right foot sweeping behind it, your left arm sweeping in front of your midsection, and your left arm sweeping out to the side. Now hop to your right, landing on your right foot and reversing the position of your other limbs. This should be a smooth, comfortable motion that mimics the movement of a speed skater in action.

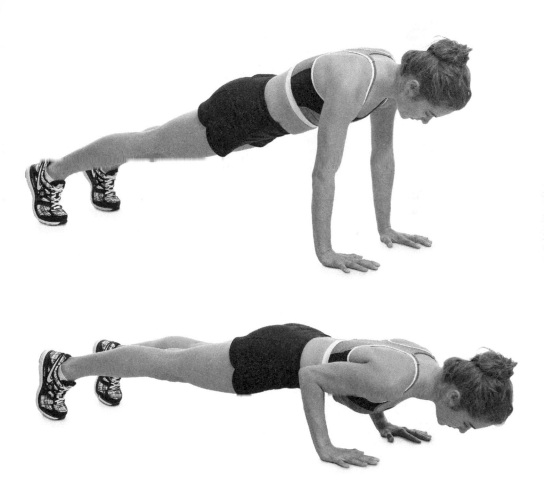

5. PUSH-UPS

■ Place your hands on the floor just outside of and below your shoulders, and straighten your arms. Keep your elbows pointing back and your arms in toward your body. Lower your chest until it almost touches the floor, then explosively push back up to the starting position.

Acknowledgments

This book would not have been possible without the support, guidance, and hard work of the following:

From David Zinczenko:

The many test panelists who tried *The Super Metabolism Diet* and saw life-changing results—and the millions of fans at eatthis.com

My brilliant co-author Keenan Mayo, who worked tirelessly to ensure this book was on the cutting-edge of metabolism, and never fell off

Marnie Cochran, an unerring editor who's never wrong

Gina Centrello, Kara Welsh, Bill Takes, Kim Hovey, Jennifer Hershey, Joe Perez, Nina Shield, Susan Corcoran, Theresa Zoro, Cindy Murray, Scott Shannon, Matt Schwartz, Toby Ernst, and Quinne Rogers at Ballantine

Michael Freidson, Jon Hammond, Olivia Tarantino, Christina Stiehl, April Benshosan, Daniel Cohen, Daniel McCarter, Charlene Lutz, Jeff Csatari, Ari Notis, JP Kyrillos, Ray Jobst, and the entire team at Galvanized Media

Ben Sherwood, Barbara Fedida, Patty Neger, and the teams at *Good Morning America* and ABC News

Jennifer Rudolph Walsh, Jon Rosen, Andy McNicol, and the astonishing talents at WME

Larry Shire, Eric Sacks, and Jonathan Erlich, who provide invaluable counsel

Elisabeth Mackey, Bella Acharya, Pamela Boyd, and the entire team at Microsoft.

Steve Lacy, Strauss Zelnick, Dan Abrams, Mehmet Oz, David Pecker, Michele Promaulayko, Dr. Jennifer Ashton, and the many friends and colleagues who are helping Americans live their Best Life

And the best family a man could ever hope for

From Keenan Mayo:

My thanks to Emily Samuel, the Mayo family, Ben and Monica Stolbach, William Langewiesche and Tia Cibani, Karen Jacob, and Jake Kestner, whose quest for healthy living and metabolic enlightenment should inspire us all.

Index

Page numbers in *italics* refer to illustrations.

About the Authors

DAVID ZINCZENKO is the *New York Times* bestselling author of *Zero Belly Diet, Zero Belly Cookbook, Zero Belly Smoothies,* and *Zero Belly Breakfasts,* the co-author of the Eat This, Not That! franchise (which has sold more than eight million copies worldwide), and the Abs Diet book series. He is a health and wellness contributor at NBC News and has appeared on *The Today Show, Good Morning America, The Oprah Winfrey Show,* and *Rachael Ray,* and is the award-winning former editor in chief of *Men's Health* and editorial director of *Women's Health, Prevention,* and *Best Life* magazines. Zinczenko is also the founder and chief executive of Galvanized Media, where he oversees a number of life-changing wellness brands. He lives in New York City.

supermetabolismdiet.com
Facebook.com/supermetabolism
Twitter: @DaveZinczenko

To inquire about booking David Zinczenko for a speaking engagement, please contact the Penguin Random House Speakers Bureau at speakers@penguinrandomhouse.com.

KEENAN MAYO is the executive editor at Galvanized Media and the editor of *Best Life.* The former editor of *Men's Fitness,* he lives in New York City.